# A Christian's Guide to Survival

# Eating To Win Beyond 2000 A.D.

*By Michael L. McCann, B.S., M.Div., Ed.D., N.D.*

I

First published 1998
by Dr. Michael L. McCann
P.O. Box 66
Cottage Grove, MN 55016
United States of America

0-9638195-1-8

Cover Art: Soon Squires

Printed and Typeset by Jerry's Impressions, Inc.
1059 South Robert Street, West Saint Paul, MN 55118 U.S.A.

# DEDICATION

This book is dedicated to the loving memory of Dr. Coy L. Purcell of Tucson, Arizona, an outstanding physician, healer and a wonderful minister of God's Word.

This anonymous saying exemplified the life of Dr. Coy Purcell who passed away recently in 1997 for his eternal home. "There is a courtesy of the heart. From it springs the purest courtesy of outward behavior." This exemplifies the life of Dr. Coy Purcell who was a true humanitarian.

# ACKNOWLEDGMENTS

I wish to express my deepest appreciation to my faithful wife Rita, who stood by me in my every endeavor to support, encourage and assist me in writing this book. I compliment her Godly patience and skill in putting this book on the computer for the final typing prior to it going to the printers. She took what needed to be done and did it, and she saw everything with the attitude that "nothing is impossible with God".

Also, I sincerely thank Mrs. Soon Squires, a dear friend and artist who did the art work for the cover of the book. God has gifted her with much talent and the work of her hands are being enjoyed by those who know excellence in the field of art.

And I want to express my appreciation to Mrs. Tina Lindstrom and Irene Cotton who devotedly spend many hours in proof-reading the first script to the last. I am very grateful for their love, kindness and willingness in this important aspect of the production of this book.

# FORWARD

*By Mrs Rita Rose McCann, B.SN*

Have you ever questioned why are there so many sick people in the Church of our Lord Jesus Christ? Why do 90 per cent of the congregation come forward for prayer to be physically healed? Isn't the Word of God powerful enough to heal those who love Him?

The Prophet Ezekiel gave us so much wisdom when he said in chapter 47:12: "And along side the torrent there will come up, along its bank on this side and on that side, all sorts of trees for food...And their fruitage must prove to be for food and their leafage for healing."

During our travels we notice the eating habits of the general population and wonder if they will survive into the 20th century. America is truly a bountiful Nation blessed by God, yet it's food is refined, processed, and void of all the nutritional elements that maintain a healthy body, soul and spirit. And when you see the farmers wearing face masks when they spread pesticides and insecticides in the spring plowing, one wonders how much of these toxic chemicals are seeping into the crops harvested in the Autumn.

This book is written to answer the questions many have on their mind: What kind of vitamins do I take and where do I get them from? It is written for everyone who wants to stay healthy and return to health and those who want to survive and win beyond 2000 A.D.

It is our desire that God's people be strong in body, soul and spirit and that they live a full life as God has promised in Psalm 91:16 "With long life, will I satisfy you and show you my salvation." Put into practice the truths you read in this book. Share it with others and be blessed!

# DISCLAIMER

Much of the advice in this book is based upon the research, professional and personal experiences of the author. If the reader has any questions concerning any material or procedure mentioned, the author strongly suggest seeking the advise of a physician or professional health care practitioner. The advice of a health care practitioner as well as proper medical screening should precede the start of any new diet, supplement or treatment program. Some of the treatments and suggestions mentioned in this book may have different effects on different people. The author is not liable for any advise, effects or consequences resulting from the use or misuse of any procedures, materials or preparations suggested in this book. The author believes that this information can be helpful to the general public.

Eating To Win Beyond 2000 A.D.

# MINISTERIAL BIBLIOGRAPHY

## Of

## Dr. Michael L. McCann

Ordained a deacon on June 6, 1972 of the Episcopal Church.

Ordained a Priest on December 21, 1972 of the Episcopal Church by Bishop A. Davis in Fort Worth, Texas.

Taught in the Bible School which he and his wife founded in England; travels the world, lecturing and teaching and praying for the sick. Dr. McCann has been given a very special Gift of Healing and a profound prophetic gift and the Word of Knowledge Ministry.

He and his wife Rita, have founded and pastored several churches during the years.

# Contents

# Contents (cont.)

# CHAPTER ONE

# THE HUMAN DILEMMA

The Twentieth Century might be called the Century of High Anxiety. People everywhere are under unusual amounts of stress causing eventual havoc with the human body. Heart disease still remains as the number one killer of our times followed by cancer and other degenerative diseases.

The human machine is a most marvelous machine which can run itself, direct itself, maintain and repair itself, and is able to do both physical and mental feats. God has so ordained that this human body is able to live to 120 years and even beyond. How do you treasure your human body? Do you keep your body in top-notch health?

Our Lord God has given us a most remarkable body. The human body is capable of incredible feats as long as it is maintained with the most essential nutrition, rest, and exercise. Yet, the average person does not have any insight into the necessary nutrition to maintain and facilitate health for prolonged periods of time.

One of the most glorious things about the human body is that it has the ability to repair itself. If you cut your finger the body begins immediately to repair the break in the tissue. If you break a bone after it has been set, the body begins to knit itself giving the added benefit of a bone stronger than before.

Even if you have neglected your body over the years, if it is given the correct nutrition, exercise, and rest it can be restored. It takes a long time to break down the body and so it takes a great deal of time to restore it.

If you have been suffering from the ills of modern society your body will need proper diet, rest, and plenty of exercise to get it back on course. You can change the state of your overall health if you are prepared to make the effort and necessary changes. So many Christians are not prepared to pay the price of good health, often times, until it is too late. They would rather be healed in a healing line rather than learn to walk in divine health. God has called us to live in divine health, but the Church of the Twentieth Century has not totally grasped this wonderful truth. We are called to live above illness. This can only be done when Christians have knowledge of nutrition, exercise, and rest so that they can enter into the divine plan.

We obtain most of our energy from food. Our food has been directly or indirectly affected by the rays of the sun. As a result, our diet must be of the utmost importance in the life of all believers.

We must maintain the quality of our blood. Pure blood circulating through the entire circulatory system must be maintained by exercise and daily physical activity.

The results of this approach to life gives the individual a powerful heart and a strong rejuvenated body which will allow the individual person to better handle the pressures of modern day living. So, as we are preparing to enter the 21st Century, if we are to be healthy, we must take charge of our own health program. It is in this manner, that we will be assured of continual good health. The Amplified Bible states in Proverbs 18:9b, "And he who does not use his endeavors to heal himself is brother to him who commits suicide". It behooves us to learn as much as we are able about proper nutrition (eating), exercise, and rest so that we reflect indwelling good health to all those around us.

Health is like freedom. You have it as long as you maintain it. Having a vigorous lifestyle and enjoying the most out of life is up to each of us. It is our responsibility to do all that we can to be in good health. Living in the Western World, our so called standard of living is supposed to be quite high as compared to the Third World. Yet, our high standard of living has not substantially reduced the rate of heart disease in this country.

We have both the power and knowledge now to change our lives from being prone toward disease to that of being most healthy. Most Christians do not know what it means to have a feeling of vigorous well being. So many of us have had that tired, worn-out feeling that we have forgotten what it means to have endless energy. We have lost that sense of well being to such a degree we settle for a "sub-level of health". It's time for all of us to raise our standards of living, learning to enjoy the best of health through proper nutrition.

The air we breathe, the water we drink, and the food we eat will either contribute to the state of health of the individual or will cause a deterioration of health. Health can only be assured if the source of our nutrition is wholesome and balanced for the needs of our particular body. This you will learn as you adopt a wholistic approach toward life. A wholistic approach toward life takes into account the spirit, soul, and body of man. These must be working in harmony with the personality to bring about that energetic state of being that all of us desire.

Our relationship with God will determine the type of mental life we will enjoy. If we are at peace with God, this in turn, will bring peace to the soul and body. This also will encourage a good mental attitude which by itself enhances a healthy body. Our attitudes are affected by the way we live each day of our lives. Daily habits can be a blessing or they can become a hindrance toward obtaining maximum health. Bad mental habits (negative thinking) can cause physical damage over the years to the human body. If you have the opportunity, just notice some of the attitudes of the chronically ill. You will be utterly amazed to find so much negative thinking among the chronically ill.

It is time to start loving your body, especially if you want to enjoy improved health. The manner in which you take care of your body is a good indication of your mental life. Many people treat their dogs better than their own bodies. The correct attitude toward health and happiness must begin by learning to love your body as God intended. If you have learned to love your body as God desires, you will enjoy an integrated relationship between your mind and body.[1]

A study done by Lester Breslow Dean, School of Public Health, UCLA, demonstrated that seven simple habits listed below will significantly influence a person's health status and life expectancy.[2] A person who practices all seven habits will enjoy a healthy life of thirty years more than the person who ignores all of them. For example, a forty-five-year-old person who practices three or less is likely to live until the age of sixty-seven. But the individual who practices all of the six habits should live to seventy-eight (based on present statistical correlations).

The following are seven simple habits that will add time and health to our lives.

1. Three regular meals a day, with few snacks.

2. Breakfast regularly.

---

1 Sukhraj S. Dhillon, Ph.D., <u>Health, Happiness, & Longevity</u>, (Japan Publications Inc. New York, N.Y., 1983), 16.

2 Ibid., 17.

3. Moderate exercise two to three times a week.

4. Moderate weight.

5. Seven to eight hours of sleep a night (not more).

6. No smoking.

7. Little or no alcohol.[3]

According to Dean Breslow's results, most people surveyed averaged two or three of these habits. It is not easy to break a habit, but with the information contained in this book, and with God's help, old habits can be replaced with new ones which will contributed to good health in your life.

## Self Examination: A Healthy Step Forward

Looking into your life introspectively is necessary if you're going to change your lifestyle. There is a genuine need for constructive assessment of your present eating habits, lifestyle, and spiritual outlook. Never allow yourself the luxury of tearing yourself down. Realize your faults and limitations without calling yourself names or expressing your frustrations in a negative way. Be positive about yourself! Your going to make a definite lifestyle change for the better. It is absolutely essential that you are positive about taking the necessary steps for a better you. It is a challenge, but one that will bring renewed strength and energy.

---

3  Ibid., 17.

In many spiritual and healing traditions, the need of prayer, coupled with a positive mental attitude, has shown to literally bring about miracles. At last, modern science has come to the conclusion that the mind can have both good and negative effect on the human body.

Start each new day with a positive affirmation about yourself. Here are just a few that I have used through the years and have proven to be most beneficial.

1. Every day and in every way I am getting healthier and wealthier.

2. My spirit, soul, and body are in perfect harmony with God.

3. My mind is clear and my body is relaxed.

4. I accept myself completely because I have been accepted in the Beloved.

5. I have new energy and strength.

6. I have become the object of Divine prosperity.

7. My life is filled with peace, power, and purpose.

These sort of positive affirmations on a daily basis will enable you to smoothly slip into a more affirmative lifestyle which will add to your new dimension of health. Change is never easy, especially changing your eating habits. Food is something that many people will not allow themselves to be deprived of for a season, nor will many alter poor eating habits.

## Facing Everyday Situations

To enjoy life to the fullest the spirit, soul, and body must be in harmony with each other. The Bible tells us in 3 John 2: "Beloved, I wish above all things that thou mayest prosper and be in health, even as thy soul prospereth". It is God's will that we be a prosperous people, but this cannot come about until we have learned how to live according to healthy principles. So many just do not know how to eat correctly for their style of life. Nor do they know how to have peace of mind which must accompany those desiring improved health.

All of us need an enthusiasm for life itself. Life goes by so fast that many never really enjoy it. Happiness and success are dependent upon our enthusiasm for living. What is your attitude each and every day? Is it drudgery for you to get out of bed in the morning? What is the first thing you think about when getting out of bed? Having a positive outlook on life will enable you to face your problems. You will release your inner energy to see solutions to your particular situation.

So many Christians do not know how to relax their minds. A few years ago the very thought of meditation would have brought some very negative comments from fundamentalist Christians. Today we now realize that there can be a Christian approach toward meditation which will bring about the inner peace and healing so necessary in our day. Just by calming the mind and focusing on the name of "Jesus" will lower blood pressure, still the thought life, and abolish worry and anxiety. This is not having a passive mind, but a mind taken over by the Peace of God which surpasses anything you can get from pills, drugs or alcohol. It is time to connect with our inner man so that we might hear the Holy Spirit as we should.

Meditation is simply a state of mind where unpleasant thoughts are blocked and concentration is focused on some pleasant thought or a word taken from Scripture. This in turn, after being practiced over a period of time, will bring incredible health blessings. Jesus promised the believer peace in this life: "Peace I leave with you, my peace I give unto you: not as the world giveth, give I unto you. Let not your heart be troubled, neither let it be afraid." (John 14:27) This is a promise from Jesus Christ but so many good Christian people just do not know how to get a hold of this precious and great promise. It is only as we learn to still our minds that we can hear the Holy Spirit and allow the troubles of an unsettled mind to finally find peace in Christ. Of course, once again, there is a price to pay. The price is your time and effort to make a lifestyle change.

As you come into this new enlightened understanding of Jesus Christ through prayer and meditation, His word will have a far more importance in your life. Your spirit, soul and body will be flowing together preparing the way for sound diet and exercise. You will become a new person with a renewed enthusiasm for life. Don't you think it's about time to consider going back to a more natural approach toward living?

Eating To Win Beyond 2000 A.D.

# CHAPTER TWO

# AN UNDERSTANDING
# OF NUTRITION

Nutrition may be defined as the process by which living organisms receive and utilize food. Nutrients are those life-sustaining constituents found within food. The average person, with the life expectancy of 70 years, who weights no more than 165 pounds, will consume about 35 tons of food in their lifetime. That is the equivalent of 16,000 bricks or enough to build two three-bedroom houses.[1] We truly need an understanding of the food we are consuming.

Whether good or bad, our eating habits are formed very early in life. Consequently, it becomes very difficult to change such habits since they are based upon both social and family traits of eating. Each of us need a knowledge of the strong relationship that exits between our eating habits and our health. This new insight will

---

1 Sukhraj S. Dhillon, Ph.D., Health, Happiness, & Longevity, (Japan Publications, Inc. New York, N.Y., 1983), 31.

assist adults in correcting their eating habits and will allow youngsters to learn at an early age a good way of eating naturally.

All human beings require food for two fundamental reasons:

1. Our food should provide the nutrients necessary for the building, upkeep, and repair of body tissues as well as those required for the essential functioning of the body.[2]

2. Food gives us the needed energy to work, play, keep basic bodily functions going, and just to live. For children and young people food is necessary to cause growth.[3]

There are approximately fifty known nutrients necessary for the functioning of the body. These include proteins (amino acids), carbohydrates (sugar and starches), fats (fatty acids), minerals, vitamins and water. No single food known to mankind contains the necessary nutrients needed for the human body.

## Proteins and Essential Amino Acids

Protein is the most plentiful substance found within the human body. It is only exceeded by water. Protein is essential for the maintenance of good health and is necessary for the growth and development of all body tissues. Muscles, blood, skin, hair, nails, and internal organs are dependent upon protein as the major source

---

2  Ibid., 31.

3  Ibid., 31.

of building materials. Protein assists in the prevention of tissues and blood from becoming too acidic or alkaline. It also assists in the regulation of the body's water balance. Enzymes, the substances necessary for basic life functions, are also formed from proteins. Antibodies assist in fighting foreign substances in the body and are also formed from protein.

Protein is used as a source of heat and energy when sufficient fats and carbohydrates are not present in the diet. Protein that is not used for body building or energy is converted by the liver and is stored as fat in the body tissues.

As digestion occurs, large molecules of proteins are decomposed into simpler units called "amino acids". Amino acids are needed for the synthesis of body proteins and other tissue constituents. Amino acids are the units from which proteins are constructed and are the end product of protein digestion.

Many of the approximately 20 amino acid molecules are able to be converted into others, or manufactured by the body if there should be a shortage of one type. There are eight amino acids which the body cannot synthesize and it is essential that they be taken into the diet in a formed structure. It is for this reason they are called "essential amino acids".[4]

Meat, cheese, milk, and eggs are considered the "protein foods". There are other sources of protein that are just as good as the above mentioned. Beans, peas,

---

4 Rudolph Ballentine, M.D., <u>Diet & Nutrition</u>, (The Himalayan International Institute, Honesdale, Pennsylvania, 1989), 113.

and soybeans have a high concentrated source of protein. Even such seeds as pumpkin and sunflower contain large quantities of protein, but it should be noted, that the essential amino acids are not found in the best ideal proportions. Grains and most vegetables contain protein, and even fruits have a small but significant amount.[5]

We in the West have the idea that only from meat, cheese, milk and eggs can we obtain sufficient protein in our diets. This is just not true. Various diets from around the world were reviewed which were based solely on grains, vegetables, and legumes with only one tenth of the protein coming from meat, milk, cheese and eggs. Nutritionists were amazed to find that a diet sufficient to supply 2,500 calories would supply about 50% more protein than needed by 98% of the population.[6]

We have now come to the conclusion, according to Dr. Rudolph Ballentine, M.D., Director of the Himalayan International Institute, that a good vegetarian diet is wholesome and healthful.[7] Western medicine now recognizes the problems of cholesterol found within meat that definitely affects the levels of cholesterol in the human serum. At the same time vegetarians do not have such high levels of cholesterol as meat eaters.[8]

---

5   Ibid., 114.

6   V. Register and L. Sonnenberg, "The Vegetarian diet", J. Am Diet Assn,(1973) 62:253-261.

7   Dhillon, Health, Happiness & Longevity, 115.

8   Ibid., 115.

We now know that the positive effects of a meat-free diet on blood cholesterol, and the possible benefits for arteriosclerosis are due to a decreased intake of fat in the diet. Though meat is high in protein, at the same time it contains a great deal of fat. Even when the fatty parts of the meat have been removed there still exists an equal amount of protein and fat. Bean and grain proteins contribute very little fat, but do bring 3 or 4 times as much complex carbohydrates.[9]

We have also learned that protein itself may have various types of effects. Vegetable protein has shown itself to have protection against arteriosclerosis as compared to the protein of animals. It is interesting to note that the Seventh Day Adventists, in some cases, are pure vegetarians; while others eat very small amounts of meat, but have significantly less heart disease and cancer as compared to other Christian groups. In addition to this, vegetarians have much lower blood pressure than meat eaters. Another significant finding is that vegetarians have less osteoporosis than those who indulge in animal flesh.[10]

There is medical evidence that the meat eaters have increased risks toward cancer of the large intestine. Vegetarians have more fiber in their diets since they eat high vegetable protein instead of meat, and this lends itself to much less diverticulosis and arteriosclerosis. It would appear that vegetable fiber absorbs a variety of environmental pollutants. These pollutants are carried

---

9  Ibid., 116.

10 Ibid., 117.

out of the body because of rapid transit of better functioning bowels.[11]

As never before in the Unites States we are being confronted with the problem of contaminated meat and meat products. This is due to the numerous pesticides being used in growing animal feed. The animal eats the feed which then stores some of the toxic poisons in its tissues. We eat the animal flesh not realizing that even cooking cannot eliminate all of the toxic waste. Thus, this toxin from pesticides is stored in human tissue, later to show itself in some form of human cancer.

Obviously, animal foods have higher concentrations of pesticides than plant foods, and the end product of these environmental toxins are being added to the diet of man. Isn't it any wonder why we have so much cancer in the United States and Western Europe?

Eating only vegetables and fruits have the capability of expelling toxins from the human body. If this is the case, than it behooves us to eat more fruits and vegetables to cleanse our bodies from accumulated toxic waste.

Foods supply carbohydrates in the human diet basically in three forms; starches, sugars and celluloses. Celluloses, along with hemicelluloses, lignin, pectin, and cutin furnish essential fibrous bulk for the human diet. It is understood that high fiber

---

11 Ibid., 117.

diets may play a significant role in cancer reduction and diseases of the intestinal tract.

The most common forms of carbohydrates are starches and sugars which are necessary for energy. These must be available in the body at all times. The average adult needs about two pounds of carbohydrates a day to maintain energy and body function. When carbohydrates are not present, body fat and protein are used as fuel. These are converted into sugars to be used as energy.

As carbohydrates are broken down by the digestive enzymes, glucose is formed and absorbed directly into the blood stream. It is used as energy to maintain bodily functions. Dairy products, which contain the sugar lactose, supply the body with a lesser amount of sugar. Plants supply most of the needed carbohydrates for human nutrition. It should be noted that carbohydrates assist in regulating protein and fat metabolism. Fats require carbohydrates for their breakdown within the liver.

Simple sugars, such as those found in fruits and honey, are readily digested. Double sugars, such as that used on the table, require additional digestive action. Starches require more digestive action before they are able to be broken down. Cellulose, which is commonly found in the skins of fruits and vegetables, is mostly undigestible and gives very little energy. Cellulose does assist in elimination since it provides a great deal of bulk. Carbohydrate snacks do give rapid energy for the body. These produce what we call a "sugar high" which causes a rapid release of insulin.

The only problem with this is that very shortly after this surge of sugar is produced in the blood stream, the blood sugar level will drop. This has often been associated with hypoglycemia and depression.

Body weight, physical activity, and basal metabolism rates will determine the amount of carbohydrates the human body will need. A lack of carbohydrates may produce ketosis, which is a condition whereby the body accumulates ketones, as a result of a deficiency or inadequate utilization of carbohydrates.[12] In addition to this, a lack of carbohydrates will cause decreased energy, depression, and will facilitate a breakdown of essential body protein.

## Fats

Fats, also known as lipids, are a highly concentrated source of energy in the human diet. After oxidation, fats provide more than twice the number of calories per gram than carbohydrates or proteins.

Fats do act as carriers for the fat-soluble vitamins A, D, E, and K. Fats assists in the absorption of vitamin D. In turn, fats help calcium to become available to body tissues especially for the bones and teeth. Fats are necessary for carotene to become vitamin A. After having eaten a fatty meal the hydrochloric acid production in the stomach is slowed.

There are two kinds of fatty acids, saturated and unsaturated. Saturated fats are hard at room

---

12 Mosby's Medical Dictionary, 4th ed. (1994), s.v. "Ketosis."

temperature. Unsaturated fats are usually liquid at room temperature. Vegetable shortenings and margarines undergo a process known as "hydrogenation". This process causes these fats to take on a more solid form of fat.

There are three "essential" fatty acids: linoleic, arachidonic, and linolenic. These are known as unsaturated fatty acids. These fatty acids are necessary for normal growth and healthy blood, arteries, and nerves. These fatty acids help keep the skin and other tissues youthful by preventing dryness and scaliness. These fatty acids assist in transportation and breakdown of cholesterol.

Cholesterol is a lipid or a fat-related substance which all human beings need for good health. Cholesterol becomes dangerous when the levels of both good and bad cholesterol are out of proper proportion, or if the level of blood serum cholesterol exceeds accepted medical levels. Apple cider vinegar and garlic help in restoring good levels of cholesterol.

Fat deficiency is very rare. The deficiency of fat will lead to eczema and other skin disorders. When extreme fat deficiencies occur it will cause severely retarded growth.

## Minerals

We hear a great deal about fats, proteins and carbohydrates, but we hear very little about minerals and the necessity of minerals in the diet. Other nutrients have stolen the lime-light in the ever existing quest to stay young and younger longer. Yet, without minerals, without their mind and body building powers, all other nutrients would be virtually useless.

Minerals, or trace elements as they are sometimes called, because they exist in such small, yet powerful amounts in the body, are required for overall mental and physical functioning. Minerals are necessary factors in maintaining proper physiological conditions and processes, such as the acid-base balance, osmotic action, elasticity and soft tissues, such as muscles.[13] Our skeletal structure's strength depends upon adequate amounts of minerals. The nerves must have them to be tranquil, strong, and vibrant. Digestion and healthful assimilation of foods depend upon the adequate "mineralization" in the digestive track. From 4 to 5 per cent of the body's weight may be considered mineral matter. Minerals are found in all tissues and fluids. They are especially obvious in the bones, teeth and cartilage.

Minerals, if in adequate amounts, will help keep the body young. There are close to 30 such minerals which help prevent premature aging by helping to preserve youthful stamina in the nerves, muscles, heart, blood, and brain. Minerals help us to have greater resistance against disease. Also, minerals give us more freedom from fatigue and greater ability to work. When individuals have sufficient minerals in their diets, they can mature, with all physical faculties to greater age, and will have a better mind than the

---

13 Carlson Wade, Magic Minerals, (Parker Publishing Company, Inc.; West Nyack, N.Y., 1968), 3.

person who suffers from single or multiple vitamin or mineral deficiency.[14]

Minerals have numerous important functions within the body. The main functions they perform are as follows:

1. The building blocks of our bodies, which is protein, is formed only in the presence of calcium, nitrogen and sulfur.

2. The entire digestive system is dependent upon potassium to cause proper function of the vagus nerve.

3. Many vitamins are totally dependent upon minerals for their functioning.

4. Minerals are necessary with vitamins to remove internal gaseous waste products. It is a fact that individuals suffering from multiple sclerosis suffer from damage to the nerve covering, caused by an excess of a carbon-nitrogen substance. It is thought that prevention of this diseased condition or removal of the harmful substance can be accomplished if the body is properly fed with minerals, especially cobalt.[15]

5. Since the insulin molecule contains zinc, and since diabetes results from an insulin shortage, it is thought that a deficiency of zinc mineral is involved with this disease.

---

14 Ibid., 3.

15 Ibid., 4.

6. Minerals influence muscle contraction and are essential for nerve response.

7. Minerals function to control body liquids and permit other nutrients to pass into the bloodstream. Without minerals other nutrients are not able to do their job as they should.

8. Blood coagulation is dependent upon mineral action. Bruises, cuts, scratches, and wounds need minerals for the healing process.

9. Personal alertness, youthful energy, and thought power all require minerals such as manganese, cooper, cobalt, iodine, zinc, magnesium, and phosphorous for utmost efficiency.

10. Minerals in our blood stream assist in creating a germ-killing action. Minerals have an antibiotic function within the blood stream provided other essential raw materials are also present.

11. Minerals are necessary for strong bones and teeth, which are composed of about 95 per cent calcium and phosphorous.[16]

Glorious health can come to us if we are eating healthy fresh food and taking needed supplements.

**Vitamins**

There is so very much written about vitamins. The information abounds and so does the misinformation. Natural vitamins are organic food substances which

---

16 Ibid., 5.

may be found in plants and animals. We know of at least twenty substances that have been discovered which are considered active in human nutrition. These vitamins are found in varying degrees in specific foods and are essential for natural growth and maintenance of good health. By in large, the body is unable to synthesize vitamins so they need to be provided in the diet or by food supplements.

Vitamins must have enzymes, which are chemical, to perform numerous necessary functions within the body. Chemical enzymes consist of two parts: one consists of a protein molecule and the other is a coenzyme. The coenzyme usually is a vitamin, or it may only contain part of a vitamin. Also, it could be a molecule which has been manufactured from a vitamin. Oxidation is the end product of enzymatic chemical action. Oxidation begins as the oxygen enters the blood stream and it travels to the cells where oxidation than takes place.

Enzymes function as catalysts. They begin the chemical reactions that allow other materials to continue their work. Inasmuch as vitamins work on the cellular level, insufficient vitamin supplementation may cause varied symptoms.

Regeneration in the body and the body chemistry often takes months. Continued vitamin supplementation will correct deficiencies within the body. Over indulgence in vitamins will cause toxicity. There are definite risks involved when there is an over-dose of vitamins.

Vitamins are described as being water-soluble or fat-soluble. The water-soluble vitamins which are the B-complex, Vitamin C, and the compounds knows as "bioflavonoids", can be measured in milligrams. The fat-soluble vitamins A, D, E, and K are measured in units known as "International Units" (IU) or "United States Pharmacopoeia" (USP).

## The American Diet

The United States of America is a land full of food. Yet at the same time, millions either are not eating correctly, or are eating all the wrong things. We have become a nation of obese people. We are also a nation of malnourished individuals who are suffering needlessly from diseases which are directly related to what we eat.

In other nations, people eat foods selected fresh from within their own natural eco-system. Here in America, from the turn of the century, our entire approach toward food and eating have changed vastly. Foods of today currently considered traditional are such things as hot dogs, Coca-Cola, Corn Flakes, Oreo cookies, Cheese Whiz, and the fast food chains across this nation. The kitchens which existed at the turn of this century have disappeared. People in America are eating less naturally than any other time in our history. Our most popular foods come from the supermarket and not the family garden. In our modern city, selecting and preparing foods are done on the basis of fashion, convenience and taste rather than on nutritional correctness. The modern American diet is usually based on taste so meat, salt, sugar, fat and artificial additives dominate our diet. These have the tendency to liven foods up which otherwise would not be palatable to the tongue. Traditional diets seek out more natural seasonings, whole grains and legumes. This than is coupled with the liveliness found in fresh vegetables. In the present day American diet, there is an excess of calories, fat, saturated fat, cholesterol, refined sugar and salt.[17] As a result of the nutritional ratio of nutrients to calories, obesity and poor nutrition have become national problems.

Americans are eating a lot of empty calories. We eat altogether too much refined white sugar, fat and refined oils. Is it any wonder that we are becoming a nation of sick people?

A healthier diet would include much less fat, less carbohydrates and more fresh fruits and vegetables. This diet would be lower in calories and would resemble a diet better related to the turn of the century when Americans lived out of their gardens.

Our teenagers in America are suffering because of the way in which they eat. They eat altogether too many prepared snacks, colas, hamburgers, french fries, malts, candies, and just plain junk food. This affects them in every area of their lives. They are sowing seeds for eventual diabetes, cancer and heart disease. It affects their behavior and can even affect their ability to learn. Attention Deficit Disorder is on the increase in America. Why? How can a child given a sugar-coated

---

17 Rudolph Ballentin, <u>Diet & Nutrition</u>, 286.

breakfast, and then later a candy bar and a glass of cola, possibly be prepared to learn? The child is on a sugar high which will cause the child not to have the strength to concentrate on his school work for any prolonged period of time. His emotional behavior will resemble his diet. If the diet is high in sugar that child will suffer needlessly because of the ignorance of the parents. Much Attention Deficit Disorder is directly related to a child's poor diet.

In developing a more wholesome diet the first step should be replacing white refined sugar with raw sugar, raw honey, natural maple sugar, molasses, sorghum, and date sugar.[18] Fresh juice is a much better drink for all the members of the family than drinking sugar-laced cola drinks. At the same time we need to make sure that we don't take in too much natural sugars because they can cause other related sugar problems. In our quest for a better diet, we need to replace white refined flour products for less refined flour products. A lot of families are making their own bread because of the new bread making machine that has been on the market, thereby controlling the ingredients of the bread. Nothing tastes better than fresh homemade bread and nothing can substitute for that delicious mouth-watering aroma. The next major change in the diet should be replacing refined vegetable oils, shortening and margarine with butterfat.[19] One must be very careful not to use too much saturated or unsaturated fats in the diet. It is

18 Ibid., 293.

19 Ibid., 294.

recommended to use only two tablespoons of butter per day.

We live in a very busy society consequently, convenience foods have found a place in our diet. They must be replaced in our quest for a better diet and health. Hydrogenated peanut butter and cheese spreads are our fourth food products to be eliminated. Also, check on the number of preservatives that are contained in a product before using it. When buying food products, be aware of those that claim to be enriched or fortified. If the item would have been left in its natural state there would be no need to put anything back into it!

When selecting food at your local supermarket make sure that nearly everything you buy is fresh. This is best of all since they will contain the highest level of nutrients especially if they have been grown organically.

There are many good sources of fresh vegetables and fruits. We need to get back to growing some of our own vegetables and planting fruit trees suitable for our climate. Getting back to nature surely will increase our health and even extend the length of our lives. Always try to have the freshest produce and don't keep the product very long in your refrigerator because you will cause a loss of nutrients. The basic nutrients can be altered and even destroyed if kept in a refrigerator too long.

Dried peas, beans and grains can be purchased at almost all grocery stores. These kinds of foodstuffs store well and travel well. While organically grown are preferred, it is not always possible to obtain them at a reasonable price. Such vegetables which are organically grown cost more because of the scarcity of land producing them.

## CHAPTER THREE

# NUTRITIONAL PHYSIOLOGY

It is most important that we have some idea of what digestion actually is. Basically digestion is that process which breaks down food into substances that will be absorbed and utilized by the body. The food will be used by the body for energy, growth, and repair.

Enzymes assist the digestive system in breaking down food substances. Enzymes are produced by the glands associated with their digestive tract. They are responsible for the chemical reactions which take place in the digestive system.

Digestion begins in the mouth as the salivary glands beneath the tongue begin to produce ptyalin, a necessary enzyme for digestion. It also breaks down carbohydrates into smaller molecules known as maltose and glucose.

Food than passes down the esophagus tube into the stomach. While in the stomach the vagus nerve produces hydrochloric acid. Then the enzyme pepsin mixes with the acid and stomach mucus to further breakdown the food chemically. Because of nerve action, ptyalin stops and a whole new series of actions are triggered off by the nerve impulses.

Nerve impulses govern the amount of stomach juices released. The presence of food and hormones are also influenced by the nerve actions.

The hormone gastrin stimulates the stomach cells to release hydrochloric acid. While pepsin is in the stomach it than is broken down into peptones. When acidity reaches a certain level, gastrin production than ceases.

As the food leaves the stomach it enters the duodenum, the first part of the small intestine. The food leaving the stomach is a thickish, acidic liquid called chyme. The duodenum produces large quantities of mucus, which protects the food from other enzymes and acid in the chyme. The duodenum receives digestive juices from the pancreas, then large amounts of bile, which have been stored in the gall bladder having been made by the liver, are than released. Bile is stored in the gall bladder until needed.

The alimentary tube is a muscular tube about thirty-three feet long. The magnificent organ starts at the mouth and ends at the anus. The canal is actually a part of two different systems. The first part of the system, the digestive system, involves the organs from the mouth to the end of the small intestine. The second part travels from the large intestine to the anus. This part of the tube is concerned with expelling waste products from the body and is part of the excretory system.

There are two hormones which trigger the release of pancreatic juices. The hormone secretin stimulates alkaline juices which than neutralize the acidic, partially digested chyme. Pancreozymin, the second hormone, causes other pancreatic enzymes to be produced. During the same time, bile is released from the gall bladder into the duodenum, thus causing the break-down of fat globules.

The pancreatic enzymes assist in breaking down proteins and carbohydrates. One of the enzymes, trypsin, aids in breaking down the peptones into smaller units called peptides. Lipase assist in breaking down fat into smaller molecules of glycerol and fatty acids. Amylase will break down carbohydrates into maltose.

The food travels down into the jejunum and ileum, and into the small intestine where the final stages of chemical changes take place. Enzymes are released from cells located in the small indentations in the walls of the jejunum and ileum. These indentations are known as the crypts of Leiberkühn.

Most food absorption takes place in the ileum. On the inner wall of the ileum are millions of minute projections called villi. Each of the villus contains a capillary and a tiny blind-end branch of the lymphatic system. This is known as a lacteal. As the digested food comes into contact with the villi, the glycerol, fatty acids and dissolved vitamins will enter the lacteals. These are than carried into the lymphatic system and are poured out into the bloodstream.

Amino acids from protein digestion, sugars from carbohydrates, vitamins and minerals, such as calcium, iron and iodine are absorbed into the capillaries in the villi. These small capillaries lead into the hepatic portal vein which then transports the food directly into the liver. Some of this is absorbed and stored in the liver while the rest passes directly into the bloodstream.

The digestive system has the task of breaking down starch-based carbohydrates, such as potatoes and bread, into individual sugar molecules. This process begins in the mouth where there is a starch-splitting enzyme called amylase which is found in saliva. Additional amylase passes down through the stomach into the intestines working on the digesting food.

Amylase breaks down starch into pairs of sugar molecules, which are then split by another series of enzymes in the small intestine. Thus only sugar molecules are absorbed into the small intestine. Eventually the sugar molecules make their way to the liver. The liver changes all the fructose and other similar compounds into glucose.

The body's mechanism makes sure that there is sufficient glucose in the bloodstream at all times. The body will either switch on or off the release of glucose from the liver. The liver stores glucose in a compound called glycogen. The muscles are used by the body to also store glycogen.

As glucose is released into the bloodstream, it is immediately taken up by the cells and insulin is released from the pancreas. Insulin, like amylase, comes from the pancreas. Insulin is produced from the islets of Langerhans and is secreted into the blood, not into the intestine.

As glucose is inside the cells, it is burnt with oxygen to produce energy. The waste products of this process is carbon dioxide and water. The carbon dioxide is carried by the bloodstream to the lungs where it is excreted back into the air. The water simply joins the pool of water which makes up about 70 per cent of the body weight.

We know that the liver stores glucose in the form of glycogen, so the energy made from burning glucose has itself to be stored in each cell to be used in small amounts to provide power for the chemical reactions on which the cell depends. The cells do this by creating high energy phosphate compounds which can easily be released for needed energy. These phosphate compounds (adenosine triphosphate or ATP is the chemical name for the compounds) can be used as energy is needed. They act like a battery because they can be recharged as needed. The recharging comes from the burning of glucose.

It is important that the glucose levels be kept on a steady level in the blood stream. If the levels are too high it produces diabetes. If the glucose level falls too low, the brain can no longer function properly. A loss of consciousness could result and this condition is known as hypoglycemia.

The blood glucose level in our bloodstream is kept constant by balancing the effect of insulin (which lowers blood glucose by pushing it into cells) with other hormones which tend to push the blood glucose up by releasing glucose from the liver. The most important hormones are adrenalin and cortisone. These both are produced by the adrenal glands. There is a growth hormone which comes from the pituitary gland in the brain which also pushes up the level of glucose.

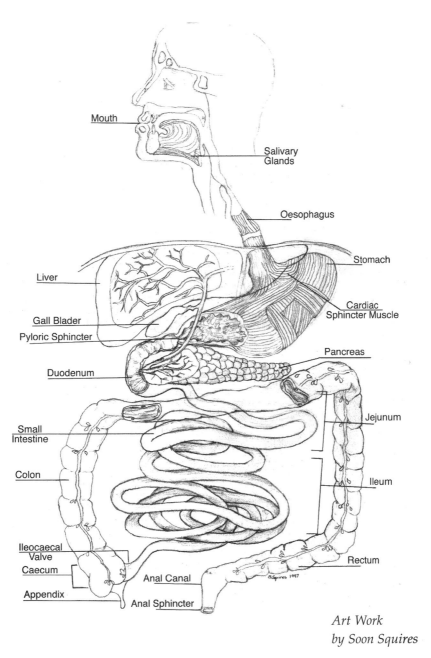

Mouth

Salivary
Glands

Oesophagus

Stomach

Liver

Cardiac
Sphincter Muscle

Gall Blader

Pyloric Sphincter

Pancreas

Duodenum

Jejunum

Small
Intestine

Colon

Ileum

Ileocaecal
Valve

Caecum

Rectum

Anal Canal

Appendix

Anal Sphincter

*Art Work
by Soon Squires*

Eating To Win Beyond 2000 A.D.

## CHAPTER FOUR

# STARTING WITH THE BOWELS - THE BIG POOP!

So many people living today have built a false concept of time. Many live 40 or even 50 years trying to figure out why they are here. After finally coming to some conclusions about life and their purpose, they find out that their bodies are literally falling apart. After having acquired countless experience and knowledge of life itself, the body tells the brain your too old and now need to prepare for your death.

As we begin to experience the ravages of premature aging coming upon us, we realize we have never taken the time to understand how long these aging processes have taken. So we begin to look for miracle cures, pills, and the latest in magnetic therapy. We find out that there isn't any quick fix-up for the problems found within our bodies. Some flock hither and yon blindly following after any guru who promises a quick fix to problems which have taken years to come about.

We become impatient to get well and want to experience youthfulness all over again but we do not understand what is involved in getting well. Mother Nature cannot be rushed. She takes her own good time based upon universal rules required for recovery.

Results are usually the same when they are not based upon natural principles of healing. The frauds take advantage of the gullible until it may be too late to receive a total recovery.

It is now time to take your health care into your own hands! By that I mean, find out what is wrong with yourself and do something positive about it. If you have been to medical doctor after medical doctor with very little or no results at all, isn't it time to try God's way of healing? That way of healing is totally natural. If you don't do something about your health today, tomorrow may be to late. Begin to change your wrong eating habits today.

Base your understanding upon knowledge. Study about natural healing and start today by putting into practice those natural healing principles.

There is no short cut to a vigorous healthy body. These things can come about but its going to take time, effort, and money. Ignorance is terribly expensive! It has taken a long time for your body to get in the shape that it is in today. One injection of the wrong stuff can relegate you to an early grave. Age is no criterion when a person is determined to get well and stay well.

We need to acquire knowledge but this new understanding must never be judgmental. We need to put into practice those things we learn so that we might turn the tide of health on our own behalf.

We must learn how to avoid degeneration in every area of our body and aim for a long range program which will encourage long life. We need to know the mistakes we made in the past and make sure we don't commit them again. It is essential that we know what damage might have occurred from eating the wrong things or doing the wrong things to our bodies. If we have this knowledge we can correct bad habits or any other incorrect pattern which has been established through the years.

Mankind, with all the vast knowledge acquired in the last fifty years, still has not truly advanced the health of the nations that much. We are slowly killing ourselves. We are plagued with illness, disease and needless suffering which was unknown a hundred years ago. It is time to learn what is necessary for good health and put into practice basic principles of good nutrition so that we might enjoy the vitality of a vigorous body.

## All Diseases Begin In The Colon

Now we come to that part of this chapter where we must really take into consideration the root cause of our health problems. All the Naturopathic Physicians, I included, believe that all diseases begin in the colon! Think about this statement a few times and you too will better understand that keeping the colon clean will assure you of a "clean bill of health". Our colon can cause endless physical difficulties that you can't even begin to imagine. If our colon has become impacted with sugars, beef burgers, french fries, white flour such as pasta, and other impacting foods, how can it possibly absorb the good we are trying to give it? We are a nation of overweight people trying to feed ourselves nutrition which can't be assimilated easily due to the impacted colon. I know this is one of the best reasons why we should practice good colon hygiene. Our colons must be kept clean from impacted fecal matter so that we might assimilate the excellent nutrition that we have a right to and that can be ours.

Although we might be Christians, it is impossible not to live in this world. Therefore, it behooves us to put into practice the things which will encourage good health. Christians ought to practice good health so that those of this world will covet what we have. You can't buy your health once its gone. Isn't it time to acquire good habits which will enhance your body's ability to live this life to the maximum?

We must be conscious of what we are eating. It is of the utmost importance that we eat natural, whole, live foods and not something that has been polluted with unnatural preservatives. Fresh fruits and vegetables are a real treat to the human body. We must eat as many fresh fruits and vegetables as possible each and every day. Cooked vegetables have very little nutritional value after being exposed to heat. Poultry, fish, legumes, whole grains, and nuts are considered to be wholesome foods. Eating live foods allows us to experience eating live enzymes. After food has been cooked the enzymes have been destroyed by the heat of cooking.

After eating foods for many years there is the problem of build-up in the intestines and colon. These must be cleaned out on a regular basis or many unwanted and unnecessary diseases will result. When I was a child my mother always cleaned our humble home both in the spring and in the autumn. This is exactly what we need to do with our bodies, but not only twice a year. Our intestines and colon need to be kept as clean as possible on a daily basis. There are times that even severe measures must be taken to clean the colon from the putrefaction of some of the food that remains on the walls of the colon. There will be times that an enema will be needed even on a daily basis for sometime to break-up the hardened fecal matter. We need to house-clean our bodies on a regular routine basis. Just as we keep the outside vegetable garden free from weeds, so we need to do "bowel gardening" to the intestines and colon of our bodies.

The concept of bowel management has not taken hold in our American culture. We just don't like to talk about our bowels as if it is something that proper people, "just don't do". How foolish this is! The idea that the bowels will take care of themselves is pure nonsense. We must have good bowel management.

Unfortunately, Americans have poor selection habits in regards to food. Not only that, it is the manner in which foods are prepared that can truly cause poor bowel function. Since we are a nation that has a phobia toward fibrous foods, the transit time of food in the digestive system is slowed causing the putrefactive bacteria to form in the bowel. These factors have been shown to be a cause of bowel disease such as colitis, diverticulitis, and other chronic disease. There is even a link toward bowel cancer when the bowels have been neglected.[1]

The colon was designed by God to be a sewage system, but by neglect it becomes a stinking cesspool of fermentation. There is an old but true saying which goes like this, "Shut your mouth, I can smell your bowels!" This kind of smell certainly gives away the diseased condition of the intestines and colon. In this state the wrong kind of bacteria will grow, setting the body up for additional disease. When the colon is clean the whole body functions better. When attention is not given to the colon it becomes filled with poisons of decay, leading to fermentation, and will cause putrefaction to enter into the blood stream.[2] This will influence the function of the brain and nervous system so that mood swings and depression become apparent from the neglect. The lungs become poisoned so that the breath becomes foul; it poisons the digestive organs so that we become distressed and bilious; it poisons the blood so that the skin looks pasty and unhealthy. Every organ of the body is affected which

---

1  Teresa Schumacher & Toni Schumacher Lund, Cleansing the Body and the Colon for a Happier and Healthier You, 9th ed. (St. George, Utah, 1994), 8.

2  Ibid.,9.

results in speeding up the aging process. We appear to be years older than we actually are. The bones and joints will pay a price for this neglect. Even our eyes look dull and the joy of living somehow has left us behind!

You and I must take responsibility for our own colon health. But not only for the health of our colon, we need to become responsible for our total well being and health. By improving the health of the bowel, this will give each of us many worthwhile benefits including more energy and vitality.

Once the bowel has been cleansed from accumulated filth and waste, the obvious next step is to give up old habits. This is the only way that we can regain health and be healthy. Health is regained when correct life giving attitudes and habits become our natural way of living. The body can be rejuvenated when it is given the nutrients we need from the food we eat. Such things as coffee and Danish pastry cannot do the job.

Colon cleansing must be something we take seriously or the results of neglect could shorten an individual's life span. A good colon cleanser may be obtained at any good health food shop. Of all the various colon cleansers, liquids, powders and pills my wife and I have tried, we have found the Herbal Fiberblend to be the very best and the very natural. This is an exclusive formulation that is available through a distributor of American Image Marketing (AIM). A colon cleanser should be taken on a daily basis, perhaps for the rest of one's life. The colon must be kept clean because it can cause untold damage to the rest of the body.

There are chemical processes which take place in the colon and they produce various gases as a by-product of bowel function. Some have no odor at all such as carbon dioxide but others like hydrogen sulfide have a pronounced odor.

Bowel gases are of no importance in a normal healthy colon. But if there is excessive gas, it is an indication of bowel disturbance and can be most serious. When there is a bowel obstruction due to constipation, the gaseous products become trapped, not enabled to leave through the anus. Extreme pressure could develop causing pain, swelling, and other bowel symptoms to appear.[3]

The production of gas in the bowel is not always the result of a normal metabolic process. Most often the production of gas in the bowel are the results of abnormal conditions. Often times the production of gas may be linked to putrefactive fermentations.[4]

If undigested protein should find its way into the colon, it will provide nourishment for unfavorable bacterial growths. The undesirable bacterial and virus hold responsibility for the breaking down of organic compounds by way of a putrefactive process. This process is undesirable due to the fact that these organisms will create toxic, poisonous, and disease-producing (morbid) by-products as a result of the metabolic function. The waste materials are most

---

3  Dr. Bernard Jensen, D.C., Tissue Cleansing Through Bowel Management, (Bernard Jensen Enterprises; Escondido, California, 1981), 46.

4  Ibid., 46.

dangerous to body tissue. These deadly organisms were never intended to inhabit the human body. The good bacteria find it most difficult to live in a dirty, toxic and constipated colon.[5]

If the bowel should have pockets, diverticulitis and ballooning, there is every indication of non-moving waste accelerating in the colon. These conditions prepare the body for fermentation, flatulence, discomfort and possible seepage of toxins into the body.

Remember a healthy colon produces very little or no flatulence, it also produces very little odor or none at all.

It is most difficult to take care of gas in the bowel. When the diet is being changed to a more natural one by using more fibrous food, patients complain of more gas than usual. This is true and will continue for even several months until the flora and fauna of the bowel have become acclimated in handling the new diet. Some patients pass off the gas easier and their stools move quickly through the colon. After a short time of several months the gas has become much less and there is very little effort in having a normal bowel movement.

If the bowel has developed diverticula, it never can be totally free of gas. Though it will be less than usual if the patient stays on his new diet, there still will be some gas forming because of the pocketing in the colon.

---

5 Ibid., 47.

One of the things we need to take into consideration here is the effect of gravity on the human body. In caring for the bowel we have both mechanical and chemical pressure to be concerned about. On the chemical side we have the effects of acidophilus bacteria, acids, and putrefactions. On the mechanical side we need to concern ourselves with the peristaltic action and the ever-present downward pull of gravity on the body. Gravity brings on more problems than most people could imagine. Gravity can be very hard on the human body.[6]

As we walk around during the course of a day the body is pulled down toward the earth. The body must contend with the constant pulling of gravity on the organs. I am convinced that if we lived on the moon we wouldn't have as many back problems as we do right now.

It has been said by Dr. Bernard Jensen that tiredness is the beginning of every disease in the body.[7] It is during the times that we are tired or exhausted that gravity has its greatest effect on the body. When we are tired, the muscles of our body begin to lose tone. Thus, the internal organs are pulled downward. Our shoulders begin to droop and other problems begin to form in the spine. Scoliosis and curvature of the spine could develop. The transverse colon is greatly effected by gravity when the body begins to lose muscle tone. The transverse colon is the only organ in the body that runs

---

6   Ibid., 48.

7   Ibid., 48.

from the right to the left side. Since the colon is made of soft tissue, a prolapse or dropped transverse can happen as the end product of the gravitational pull.[8]

Illness and disease are states of disquietude within the body. Remember we talked about the need of harmony within the spirit, soul, and body. When disease breaks out, there is a disharmony, a disquietude within the human organism. It's sense of peace and ease has been disturbed which will effect the entire human make-up of the person.

One of the subtlest forms of disharmony within the human organism is the chemical or nutritional imbalance. It is often overlooked by many good medical doctors since it may be related to a chronic condition. I like all of my patients to have a hair biopsy. From this we are able to know exactly what chemical imbalances are present within the body. After this knowledge has been obtained, we then can proceed with a proper nutritional program to bring the imbalances back to the level they should be within the human organism. So many diseases are related to chemical imbalances.

When toxic substances in the colon seep into the body's tissues, it's like having someone poison you without your knowledge of what they are doing. Arsenic administrated over a prolonged period of time in small doses will eventually kill the person. It is the same with the toxic waste matter in the colon; eventu-

---

8  Ibid., 48.

ally it will cause disease and perhaps even death. The toxic waste matter will wear down the resistance and the health of body tissues of all major organs.[9]

Mankind is living in a toxic, poisonous polluted environment. I just recently came back from Europe where, to my utter amazement, the Europeans have done very little to clear up the air in their major cities.

Our food, water, and the air we breath is polluted. Look at the meat recall by Hudson's Food this past summer. The company had to recall 25 million pounds of hamburger because of the fear of E. Coli infection. Just what does this mean for all of us? It means we are going to have to be extremely careful in buying and using the products which we find at the market since they could be deadly.

People today are more toxic than at any other time in recorded history. The amount of toxicity is a nightmare for all of us since we are all involved in one way or another. The need to detoxify and cleanse the body is so absolutely necessary. Many of the people that come into contact with me are laden with toxicity. The first thing that we have to do is to clean out their colons, so that colon health may bring health to the rest of the body.

Man is a human spirit. He is spirit, soul, and body. If his body is not in balance nothing else will be in balance either. Perhaps this sounds rather harsh but it is not intended to be. It is our job to restore balance

---

9    Ibid., 59.

back to the body. When we begin this process, I tell my patients it took you a long time to get this way and is going to take quality time to restore health to your broken down human organism. Remember when the bowels fail, you are in a terrible predicament. Metabolic shock waves will effect every organ in the body.

As we clean the body and remove the toxic poisons and feed the body with the necessary appropriate nutrition, the body will respond positively. Only then will we see the reversal of disease, and health will come back to the body. It starts with the colon!

We so abuse our colons by not taking care of them. Dr. Bernard Jensen, an authority on colon hygiene, tells us that the bowel wall needs sodium which will neutralize the acids. The average person will produce much acid in his body and in turn this will draw sodium out of the body. In addition to sodium, the bowel needs potassium since it acts as a muscle strengthener. Most of us do not realize the unique task of potassium which neutralizes acids. The body will take potassium from the bowel walls when there isn't sufficient potassium in the diet. Consequently, the bowel functions in a semi-starvation state for the needed chemical for day to day living. The most important minerals must be present in our diet or the bowel will suffer needlessly.[10]

---

10 Ibid, 60.

A healthy bowel should contain sodium, potassium, and magnesium for proper functioning. Unfortunately, these three necessary elements are lacking greatly today in our lifeless foods. Sodium is a chemical element which functions as a neutralizer and it is also found in the lymphatic system. It is needed by those body tissues that are pliable, active, and movable such as the joints, ligaments, and tendons.[11]

Magnesium is known as the great relaxer especially for the bowel. It is essential for good bowel movements. Magnesium may be found in salad vegetables and is abundant in yellow corn. Corn meal is another source of magnesium. Corn bread contains this element but not to the degree it did fifty years ago. Corn meal is highly refined but still contains some magnesium.

Lasting health can only come as we learn to discipline ourselves on a daily basis. A daily effort of cleanliness of body, mind, and spirit will bless us with lasting results. If there isn't a consistent effort on our part to change our life styles, we will never know the benefits of lasting health.

As the body becomes polluted with toxic waste substances, those forces which maintain health and vitality become diminished. To the degree that the body is polluted, the intestinal flora suffer in proportion to the invasion of filth. The end product of this is disease.

---

11 Ibid., 61.

Intestinal flora are those micro organisms which live within the human bowel.[12] There are numerous forms of microscopic life living within the colon. Some of it is very good while others are most dangerous if they are the predominate form of microscopic life. When health is in abundance, we will see a greater proportion of the good bacteria living within the bowel.

According to Dr. Bernard Jensen, the flora in the bowel determines the state of health in an individual. He describes the bowel as the mobile compost heap constantly giving up finished compost and taking on new materials for treatment.[13]

A compost heap is a most interesting thing. It is there that we throw away the waste products of living things. Things are placed there such as old pumpkin rinds, watermelon rinds, corn cobs, old leaves and the list goes on. These in time will undergo total transformation. When the process has been finished we have the best fertilizer that could possibly be found. From the death of things comes life for new beginnings.

The bacterial flora act as recyclers or transformers. They are the work force of the bowel. They perform some of the most advanced chemical operations known to mankind. They live within the large colon. It is estimated that the colon contains about 400 to 500 varieties of bacteria, fungi, yeast, and virus. At the same time, the population of these will vary from the top of the colon to the bottom and from side to side.

---

12 Ibid., 64.

13 Ibid., 65.

Medical research has shown that the mucus secreted by the intestines will determine the kind of bacteria that will grow there. It is now understood that it will take about a year after there has been a dietary change to alter the status of the bacteria found in the colon. Drugs especially will change the climate of bacteria in the bowel.

We have found that the "broad spectrum" antibiotics will kill both the good bacteria and the bad. Also, individuals taking antibiotics have shown to have high levels of cholesterol. The bacteria which help control blood cholesterol are killed off by antibiotics. If antibiotics are frequently used the body will build an immunity against them. When there is a genuine need for them the body may not be able to respond to the drug. It's best not to use antibiotics but only in the greatest of need.

The bowel needs the good kind of bacteria. We have found that lactobacillus acidophilus thrives in sour milk. The bacterial action in the milk produces a chemical reaction which breaks down the milk substance, and makes them an ideal food for the bowel. The bacteria that we want in the colon are lactobacillus, acidophilus, bulgaricus, brevius, and saliveria. Most of these can be found in natural yogurt and sour milk. Be very careful when buying yogurt since today many manufactures are using aspertain in place of sugar. Try to purchase natural yogurt without the added chemical found in other brands.

As we are trying to provide a good environment for acidophilus, we will begin to eliminate the bacillus coli. The bacillus coli is a very negative bacteria which can cause great harm if it gets out of control.

When a child is breast fed from birth until the time of weaning, the child will have his colon totally established with the good bacteria. Cow's milk does not contain colostrum which the mother's milk certainly does. Colostrum aids in the peristaltic action of the child's bowel. The colostrum helps establish an acid base for the colon which is what is desired.

If the child's colon becomes acid in nature, aided by breast feeding, then the acidophilus will multiply rapidly and literally flourish. If the colon is alkaline in nature the opportunity for bacillus coli will be encouraged. This bacteria will cause problems down the road if not kept in check.

Children who have been breast fed have less problems with disease later on during their growth periods. We also know that children who are breast fed have less epilepsy than those children who were not breast fed.

We are able to find the good kinds of bacteria in soured milk. Sour milk is also known as turned, fermented, curdled, and clabbered milk.[14] It is known by the Bulgarians and Turks as yogurt. The Russians call it Kefir.

If we are to be effective in colon hygiene we need to eat those foods that are very high in lactobacillus

14 Ibid., 70.

acidophilus. Lactobacillus is a member of the aciduric lactobacillus group which can easily be found in nature.

Having a clean bowel and bowel cleansing is a most important element in any lasting program of natural healing. It is essential that toxic waste be removed as soon as possible to prevent any further downward spiral of ill health.

Our colon cleansing program must have the following elements involved in it to be most effective:

1. the colon must be kept clean by removing toxic waste and accumulated fecal matter;

2. the diet must be changed to an elimination and cleansing diet;

3. a 24 hour fast once a week;

4. colonic irrigation by enemas or colonic flushing;

5. and changing our mental attitude to a more positive one. This may sound like a great deal to do, but we do a little bit at a time.

I would encourage you to go to a good health food shop and purchase a book about bowel cleansing. This will enable you to know the proper procedure in giving yourself an enema or seek out a colon hygienist.

The colon is the most important organ in the body. As you give it the proper respect, it will add years to your life. Your body will become younger and healthier as you keep the colon clean from wastes and toxins which would have eventually brought pain, disease and suffering. These toxins that are being discarded are saving you from more serious diseases. Be happy you are paying your bill now in a less costly way!

Eating To Win Beyond 2000 A.D.

# CHAPTER FIVE

# SUGAR AND CANDY AND MY ACHING SWEET TOOTH

This chapter is on the negative effects of the use of white sugar as it is found in foods, candy, and even pastries. At last some people in the United States are wakening up to understand how devastating sugar actually can be. Diabetes has made such a terrible inroad to our modern society. It is time to warn the nation of this horrific plague that will cause needless suffering and pain.

The warning that is being heralded across America is not being heeded by the population. It is as if the warning goes into one ear and out the other. People will not take counsel until they have been struck with diabetes. Then the warning may be too late since they may have to suffer the effects of insulin injections and the loss of health.

When sugar is eaten in any form, in food or in liquids like colas, it ferments in the stomach and intestines and produces acetic acid, carbon acid, and alcohol.

Acetic acid is used by physicians to burn warts off of human skin. It is destructive and a powerful acid which should be used with the greatest of discretion. If this acid is so destructive on the outside of the body, what do you think that it will do to the intestinal tract? This acid penetrates the system with great rapidity and acts on the nerves of the intestinal tract with paralyzing consequences.[1]

As alcohol is also produced when white sugar is eaten in candy or other foods containing sugar, it has an even more destructive effect on the body. When alcohol is formed in the human body, it acts as a solvent for elements which are only soluble in alcohol. This drug tends to destroy the texture of the kidneys.[2] Alcohol produced from eating sugar functions in a similar manner as drinking alcoholic beverages. The nerves which are closely related to the brain are disrupted, so concentration and locomotion are disturbed just as if one is drinking alcoholic beverages. Naturally this process is a much slower rate than drinking beverages containing alcohol.

When we eat white sugar, or drink liquids containing it, the response of the pancreas is shocking. The pancreas, the most active of our digestive glands, is negatively affected. It secretes its insulin directly into

---

1 Dr. N. W. Walker, D.Sc., **Become Younger**, (O'Sullivan Woodside & Company, Phoenix, Arizona, 1984), 44.

2 Ibid., 45.

the duodenum allowing us to digest several different kinds of food at the same time. The pancreas literally goes into high gear trying to deal with the white sugar which has been ingested. It suffers needlessly since we are the ones who should know better than eating anything with sugar. The pancreas is overworked and placed in the position of exhaustion. White sugar is a highly processed dead food with no positive nutritional value. It is the cause of many sicknesses and afflictions. Sugar is a drug in the human system, and people who constantly use this drug find it most difficult to give up.

When we speak of the destructive effects of sugar, we are referring to the manufactured product. In the category of sugar, we include white, brown, raw, and every other kind including molasses and maple sugar since they all have been processed with intense heat. White sugar is perhaps the most destructive since it is usually refined with the use of sulfuric acid.[3]

The healthiest sugars that actually benefit mankind are the natural sugars found in raw fruits and honey. All fruits and many vegetables, when raw, contain natural sugars known as fructose. The American Dental Association knows how harmful sugar can be to the teeth of children. When children are allowed to eat candy in any form, this will eventually affect their teeth causing needless decay. It has been determined that the use of white sugar over the years will cause pyorrhea. Pyorrhea is the product of the insidious,

---

3  Ibid., 45.

slow degeneration of the gums and teeth due to excessive use of white sugar and sugar products.[4] Starch foods do play a small role in this process but sugar is the major culprit.

Sugar is not only harmful in itself, but when it is coupled with fruit it destroys their nutritional value. Thus, they become almost worthless as a good source of fructose. Fruits are an excellent cleansers of the bowels and those which are acid to the taste produce an alkaline reaction in the system. However, when sugar is added, the chemical reaction of the digestion is altered. The end product is excessive acids in the body.

If we are to be healthy, all sugars must be avoided. White sugar is most harmful to the human body. Those that are found in foods should be avoided as those found within colas. Candies and sweets must become a thing of the past if we are to rejuvenate our bodies.

When there is a need to have something sweet, try using natural honey which has been extracted from the honeycomb and has not been processed by heating it. Honey is a pre-digested sweet or carbohydrate. This is excellent when put on fruits. The fructose is not altered by the use of honey.

Have you ever tried dates, or figs, raisins or other fruits rich in natural sugar? You will be surprised how good these can be for you if you have a sweet tooth.

---

4  Ibid., 46.

There is so much advertisement about eating certain candy bars which supposedly provide a great deal of energy. There is a partial truth to this claim. When the candy bar has been consumed, the blood sugar level soars for a period of about 20 to 30 minutes. Then the blood sugar level drops substantially as insulin does its job. If this is repeated over and over the person becomes "depressed" as a result of lowering the blood sugar level.

It is most important that we use our intelligence before eating anything with white sugar in it. Think carefully about giving up white sugar. Of course, it maybe a struggle for some of you but the battle is worth it. Your health will improve.

In 1900 the American population ate about 10 pounds of sugar per person per year.[5]

The need of calcium is absolutely essential as we grow older and it must be provided. The problem with many people is that they don't know that sugar drains the bones of needed calcium. Perhaps this is one reason we see so many older people bent over from a calcium deficiency.

We also know that sugar and sugared foods cause a B-1 deficiency. When this has become extreme, a state of depression is produced by this shortage and the

---

5  Bernard Jensen, Ph.D., <u>Food Healing for Man</u>, (Bernard Jensen Enterprises; Escondido, California , 1983), 44.

individual may even become suicidal. We need to avoid sugar like the plague.[6]

We are now aware of the fact that sugar can upset the calcium metabolism in the body and could lead to glandular imbalances.[7] We know that food products are loaded with sugar. When white sugar and white flour are combined these two will lead to a prevalence of numerous diseases.

Dental research shows that cavities are commonly a sign of calcium deficiency due to a glandular imbalance as the result of excessive sugar consumption.[8] Sugar intake is up by 135 pounds per individual annually.[9] Could this not account for the poor dental health that we are enjoying?

Our country is starving for calcium. Sugar, and its use, actually effects the body to surrender calcium from its own tissues. Thus, it deprives the growing bone structure as well as the teeth of the necessary calcium needed for normal function and growth.

My wife and I have visited West Africa on several occasions and admired the beautiful teeth in the African people. Their generous smiles shine forth the clean straight white teeth that God has given them. Then we noticed that the women especially walked with their backs straight and without any curves in

---

6  Ibid., 104.

7  Ibid., 140.

8  Ibid., 164.

9  Ibid., 164.

them. Sugar is not plentiful in West Africa as it is in the West. The diseases of the Western Culture do not plague the Africans to the extent that we are plagued. They do not suffer the many ailments that we in the West have to guard against. Yet, we notice that when the individual African moves to Germany, England or America, and takes on that country's eating habits, the same symptoms of the citizens of those nations are now being manifested upon them. I believe that sugar is truly a poison that must not be part of our diet.

Too much sugar will eventually harm every organ of the body. Sugar is first stored in the liver in the form of glycogen and later stored as fatty acids. When it is stored as a fatty acid it will be stored in the least exercised part of the anatomy. Later it attacks the kidneys and heart. The nervous system, lymphatic, and circulatory systems are also attacked by sugar as well as all body tissues. The immune system looses its resistance against germs and bacteria and becomes generally impaired in its ability to function. There also will appear a loss in the most valuable B-complex vitamins.[10]

Refined white sugar can be linked to heart ailments, diabetes and cancer. When refined white flour is added with sugar, it becomes a lifeless devitalized food making up the majority of the diet eaten in the United States.

It is now necessary to make a decision. Can you afford to continue to eat white sugar? Your health is at

---

10 Ibid., 170.

stake. You will not win by eating this deadly product which is devastating to the human body. Throw your sugar bowl out. Change your eating habits and you will win beyond 2000 A.D.

## CHAPTER SIX

# THE NATURAL DIET OR LET'S BECOME VEGETARIANS

The whole idea of vegetarianism to many good Christians is totally repugnant. They cannot conceive of not eating meat. Yet, today there are so many good reasons not to eat animal flesh. Perhaps the main one is the fact that animals raised today have been treated with both hormones and antibiotics. By the way, antibiotics are given to farm animals on a regular basis which then enters the food chain which we consume. Many of these drugs survive the cooking process and then enter our bodies. It is the same with the hormones being used to cause chickens to have larger breasts. We eat those products without realizing the danger that they might present to our bodies.

The consumption of excessive meat and processed foods causes us to have an unbalanced diet but can even raise havoc in our systems. Meat contains a great deal of protein but is completely lacking in carbohydrates, fiber, calcium, and other health promoting vitamins. These missing vitamins may be obtained from fresh vegetables, fruit, grains, and dairy products. A balanced vegetarian diet can supply all of the nutrition that is needed by the human body. Vegetarians enjoy very good health. They have much less heart disease and cancer than meat eaters. Vegetarians live longer than non-vegetarians. There are several excellent examples of longevity found amongst the Hunzans of Pakistan, the Abkhasians of Russia, and the Vilcbambams of Ecuador. These people eat very little meat and in most cases none at all. We do know that the level of exercise and the absence of stress has greatly aided these peoples in living longer. We know now that the "secret" of their natural diet has been proven by medical evidence and the scientific world. Only in the last ten years has there been an emphasis on the need of additional fibre and raw vegetables and fruit in the diet.

A natural diet consists of wholesome foods which have been grown organically (preferably) or resembling the natural state as close as possible. These foods are not processed or preserved with chemicals. They would include brown rice, whole wheat and fresh vegetables and fruits, which should be eaten raw and not cooked. Foods of this nature are low in fats, cholesterol, protein and highly refined carbohydrates. White sugar is not part of this diet, neither are canned fruits and vegetables part of a good vegetarian diet. Eating this way will bring about the desired weight that is perfect for your body. There will be little fat and no sugar in the diet, so naturally, there should be a good reduction in weight.

By in large Americans have become accustomed to eating convenience foods, so it might be somewhat difficult at first to be on this most excellent program of natural eating. Once the diet has been tried for several weeks, the improvement in health and the added benefits of weight loss will commend the diet as a permanent way of life. The diet may be approached in a step by step fashion. In this manner you start eliminating foods from your diet and add natural foods one step at a time.

Natural foods are much better for our bodies than foods made popular by the big food companies. These kinds of foods popularized for their convenience and quickness do not possess the qualities that live foods contain.

A natural diet of wholesome foods and dairy products comes close to a good vegetarian diet. Vegetarians who eat fruits, vegetables and dairy products are called lactovegetarians. Those vegetarians who eat eggs are known as lacto-ovo-vegetarians. Those vegetarians who eat only fruits and vegetables are called vegans vegetarians. Vegetarians are far healthier than those who consume animal flesh. Do you think that becoming a vegetarian is something to pray about?

A vegetarian diet reduces the risk of heart attack and stroke substantially. A diet rich in animal flesh does not commend itself to a healthy heart. It has now been shown that vegetarianism lends itself to a longer life.

Some vegetarians truly love raising their own food without using chemicals or nitrate type fertilizers. Some become vegetarians because they deplore the killing of animals. Others adopt this lifestyle because their digestive system just cannot handle meat. Still others become vegetarians for religious reasons. The Seventh Day Adventists in America are noted for their long life and healthy life style.

Unprocessed vegetarian foods are low in fat and cholesterol. A close examination of these foods show that they are high in carbohydrates and fiber with an abundance of natural vitamins and minerals.[1] It is not that difficult to become accustomed to vegetarian protein. It truly is as satisfying as meat protein.

As we look through the centuries we find that the hardiest, longest living people in the world were active vegetarians. President Thomas Jefferson was a semi-vegetarian who lived to be eighty-three years of age. He wrote, "I have lived temperately, eating little animal food, and not as an aliment, so much as a condiment for the vegetables which constitute my principal diet."[2] Others who adopted a similar lifestyle were George Bernard Shaw, Leonardo de Vinci, Ralph Waldo Emerson, Henry David Thoreau, Benjamin Franklin, Mahatma Gandhi, Albert Schweitzer, and Gloria Swanson.[3]

---

1 Sukhraji S. Dhillon, Ph.D., "Health, Happiness & Longevity", (Japan Publicatiions, Inc. 1983), 79.

2 Ibid., 80.

3 Ibid., 80.

The beauty of a vegetarian diet is that it is economical. Meat is very expensive and is not that efficient in supplying the proteins that we need. It is far more practical to use our land for growing food for human beings than for feeding animals which will shortly be slaughtered for their flesh.

We truly must make choices concerning our diet and longevity. Let's all cut down on the amount of meat that we eat and start eating more vegetables and fresh fruits.

With the ever increasing population world-wide, we need to seek other sources of protein which does not come from meat. Such countries as China and India have for hundreds of years been eating more vegetable protein than animal protein. As our world becomes more and more populated we will be forced to use more soybean products since they are easy to grow and are most beneficial to the human body.

The vegetarian diet provides an additional advantage of "eating low" on the food chain The higher we eat on the food chain the risks of acquiring more toxic material becomes apparent. Vegetables and fruits do not have the toxicity that meat possesses.[4] Vegetarianism is just good for all of us. You will begin to enjoy the best of health as you eat less meat or no meat at all. Remember that chicken and fish are still meat.

For whatever reason people become vegetarians the benefits are absolutely outstanding. It is known that

---

4   Ibid., 82.

vegetarians have a higher rate of endurance than meat eaters.[5]

It is an interesting scientific fact that carnivores have a comparatively short smooth intestinal tract, only about three times the length of their bodies. Carnivores digest their food more rapidly than herbivores. Man's intestinal tract is about thirty feet long indicating that man's digestive tract is more suitable for vegetables and fruits than meat. The rate of colon cancer among meat eaters is of a much higher rate than vegetarians. Perhaps this is due to the fact that the waste stays longer in the bowel. A carnivore eliminates more rapidly than herbivores.[6]

Early generations of mankind required meat at times in order to survive. Scientific analysis of fossilized human fecal matter shows that they subsisted mainly on vegetation. Fruits, nuts, tubers, berries, and grains were found in the fecal matter. Therefore, we may safely assume that early man was almost vegetarian if not totally vegetarian. With the onset of agriculture and the knowledge of cultivation of crops for food, this assured early man a continuous supply of vegetables and fruits. It was much later that man domesticated animals for food. It is thought that domesticated animals were suppliers of such foods as milk and eggs. Biologically man is constructed more as a vegetarian, and not as a consumer of large quantities of animal flesh.

---

5   Ibid., 82.

6   Ibid., 83.

In the United States we have an over emphasis on protein consumption. There has been skepticism about the vegetarian diet since many believe that they will not get enough protein on this diet. You will be able to have enough protein as you learn to eat a balanced diet. A vegetarian diet can supply all the necessary nutrients to sustain a high quality of life. It does not matter if you are a vegetarian or not, what is important is that you get the needed nutrients to meet your nutritional need.

If one wants to adopt a vegetarian diet it is best that they spend some time learning how to combine beans and rice together. There are excellent combinations which will provide more than enough protein from these foods. There is a need for knowledge and understanding of putting the right foods together for both protein supply and all other nutritional requirements.

The vegetarian diet can be used as a means of prevention of disease. It is a known fact that many health problems are the result of the accumulation of poison through improper eating and a steady intake of meat which can only make matters worse. Fresh juices made from vegetables and fruit juices are most healthful for those who suffer from chronic disease. Juicing on a daily basis is perhaps the best thing anyone can do for their bodies. Juicing provides the live enzymes that we need to improve our health and even the quality of life.

There are times when we will feel uncomfortable by drinking fresh juices. The reason for this is that toxins are leaving the body, and there will be different symptoms from light headedness to even diarrhea.

Fasting is another excellent method of riding the body of toxins and poisonous matter. Fasting during a sickness can have a most positive effect in overcoming the illness. Fasting permits the digestive system to rest while at the same time forcing the body to use reserved sources of fat. Today we are so orientated to use drugs to suppress pain that it just adds more poison to the human system. In many instances taking recommended drugs can be a source of great toxins and poisons which later will result in some other disease. Doctors in Europe now realize that fever may have the effect of activating the antibodies that help fight against the invading bacteria or virus. By using aspirin we can reduce the fever and dull the pain, but the source of the problem will still be there and eventually will break out in some other disease later on.

As we have discussed earlier, cancers of the colon, breast and uterus are very rare amongst vegetarian groups such as the Seventh Day Adventists in comparison to meat eating individuals. Such vegetables as cauliflower, broccoli, turnips, cabbage, spinach, celery, citrus fruits, beans and seeds actually stimulate the body to produce anti-cancer enzymes.[7]

Another observable trait of vegetarianism is the effect of greater bone density among older persons and a lower incidence of osteoporosis and its related complication.[8] Perhaps this is the result of a lesser acid

---

7  Ibid., 90.

8  Ibid., 90.

residue in the body causing the body to draw less calcium from bone stores.

Natural foods eaten raw are an excellent source of roughage or fiber for the intestinal tract. There is a definite correlation between fiber that is eaten on a daily basis and the rate of heart attacks and digestive problems. We must pay attention to our daily need of fiber because it is so very essential.

Fiber comes from the cell wall of the plant which adds roughage or bulk to our diet. By in large, fiber is not digestible except for the smallest amounts broken down by the intestinal bacteria. A chemical analysis of fiber shows us that it is made up of cellulose, hemicellulose, lignin, pectin and cutin.[9] The amount of these that we would eat is dependent upon the plant itself and how it was grown. Fiber may be found in grains, fruits and vegetables.

The benefits of fiber are numerous, such as preventing constipation, diverticulosis (a disease which causes pouching along the intestinal tract especially the colon), and cancer. Fiber does soften the stools and it does affect the bulk of the feces causing a speedy transit through the intestines. A high fiber diet causes quicker transit time through the bowels, thus allowing less time in the colon for bacteria to produce cancer causing agents.

It has been said that eating too much fat is a factor in colon cancer. If that is true, eating fiber and a low fat diet should help prevent cancer from forming in the

---

9  Ibid., 91.

colon. We also know that a high fiber diet helps in lowering cholesterol. The end product of this is decreased heart disease. We have found that eating about 7 ounces of carrots at breakfast for three full weeks could possibly lower cholesterol as much as 11 percent and increase the amount of fat excreted by 50 percent.[10] It is thought that the ability of the fibers to lower cholesterol may result from its propensity to stimulate the excretion of bile acids, which are made from cholesterol. It has been shown that fiber helps lower blood pressure.

People who consume meat and processed foods need to incorporate more fiber into their diets. Fiber does cause gas. Intestinal gas is the by-product of fiber for several weeks until the colon has produced the needed bacteria to handle the change of your diet. Intestinal gas is only temporary and will subside naturally as your colon welcomes this positive change of diet.

Dieting just does not work. How many times have we all tried to take pounds off and did so only to see them come back after a few months? A vegetarian diet is a wonderful way in which to reduce your body weight while still enjoying eating an excellent diet. You don't have to starve on a non-meat diet.

There are many side effects from being on a weight reduction program. There is the stress and the continual desire of wanting something to eat. The problem of over weight in America is almost epidemic. Obesity is

---

10 Ibid., 92.

a major problem in this country. I am surprised that more people haven't tried vegetarianism. Undoubtedly it is the lack of information and awareness about vegetarian nutrition that keeps people back from trying it. Eating simple, low fat, low calorie food of which most comes from plants will help you in losing weight. The body will respond by feeling better and even lighter as you pursue this dietary change. Vegetables are low in calories, but high in natural vitamins and minerals.

Let's take a look at a good vegetarian meal. The meal may consists of 5 ounces of kidney beans, green beans and fresh vegetables, and a slice of dark rye bread. This doesn't even come to a 5 ounce steak dinner in caloric consumption. A 5 ounce steak has over 500 calories in it and if you eat a baked potato, salad, bread and a desert, you have eaten almost 3000 calories in that meal. While in the vegetarian meal, you have just over a thousand calories. You will begin to lose that weight on a permanent basis and not suffer the hunger associated with dieting.

On the vegetarian diet your cholesterol will come down naturally without the need of drugs. Your blood pressure will be normal for your age group. You will look younger and feel ever so much better. Isn't it time to pray about being a vegetarian?

When you look carefully at the vegetarian diet, we see that fruits and vegetables contain about 80 percent water. So it is normal for many people to lose weight on this diet of fruits and vegetables. A vegetarian diet is bulk and most filling. It is most difficult to eat more calories than your body will actually burn. The end product is weight loss for those who start eating vegetarian. So not only is it more healthy but the added benefit of weight loss and weight maintenance encourages people who have had a weight problem in the past.

Learning how to cook vegetables can be more enjoyable than that of cooking meats. The variety of taste found in the vegetable kingdom is vast. Learn how to select your protein needs by choosing legumes such as soybeans along with cereals and milk for obtaining the necessary amino acids.

As we are learning about meat eating and how it can be detrimental to health, we now must learn about vegetarian cooking and foods. Without any doubt, vegetables rank high among the best constituents of a good diet. As we chose our food more selectively we will need less vitamin and mineral supplementation since we will be getting enough from our new diet.

The understanding of a good diet begins with taking (1) bread and cereal group (about four servings); (2) protein group - nuts and legumes (about two servings), (3) fruit and vegetable group (five servings), (4) milk group (about two servings for adults; children and teenagers need much more).[11]

If we will take the time and make the effort to learn how to eat as a vegetarian, it can only be beneficial.

---

11 Ibid., 96.

Your body will undergo great changes which will bring renewed health and stamina. If we are going to win in being healthy, there must be a decision to eat less meat or no meat at all. I am not trying to convert anyone to a vegetarian diet but just show you the benefits and let each person decide for themselves.

Eating To Win Beyond 2000 A.D.

# CHAPTER SEVEN

# STAYING YOUNGER LONGER

According to the National Institute of Aging, the signs of aging are those physical and behavioral changes which will occur at predictable periods of time during the life of any individual.

In human beings some predictable signs of aging are: changes in lung capacity and the expansion of the chest; bone loss; the pupil in the eyes become smaller; sleeping disorders occur; a change in the glucose tolerance is noted; the weakening of the immune system; cardiovascular changes and both hearing and sight changes take place.

One of the most important indications of aging is a decreased lung capacity and chest expansion. This is an indication of declining health and aging. The ability to inhale and the amount of air expelled declines gradually over the years. This could possibly be the result of change in the lung walls. The primary function of the lungs is their ability to inhale oxygen and expel carbon dioxide. Usually the right lung is larger than the left since it has three lobes while the left has two. As we inhale the inspired air reaches the alveoli and is distributed evenly to the millions of alveoli in the lungs. As oxygen and carbon dioxide pass across the alveolar capillary membranes the blood flow is distributed evenly to all the ventilated alveoli.[1]

After forty years of age the basal metabolic rate, our oxygen consumption, slowly declines. When one reaches 80 years of age there is a very rapid decline which becomes apparent. As a result of a slower metabolic rate older people become tired more easily. Breathing exercises on a daily basis will help our lungs keep their oxygen capacity at normal levels.

As we begin to grow older somewhere between the ages of 40 and 45, many of us suffer great changes in our vision. Because of changes in the pupil and the lens, less light is available to the retina. The retina of a 20 year old individual may receive three times as much light as the retina of a 40 year old person. Numerous studies have been done about this condition but still we are in doubt why this happens.[2]

Farsightedness is another vision-related sign of aging. So many need glasses between the ages of 40 and 45. We suffer from the inability of not being able to

---

1   Ida G. Dox, Ph.D., B. John Melloni, Ph.D., and Gilbert M. Eisner, M.D., The Harper Collins Illustrated Medical Dictionary, (Harper Collins, New York, N.Y., 1993), 254 .

2   Sukhraj S. Dhillon, Ph.D., Health, Happiness, & Longevity, (Japan Publications, Inc., New York, N.Y., 1983), 114.

focus on near objects. This is due in part from changes in the lens and the muscular forces acting upon it.[3]

Bone loss is something that we are hearing a great deal about today. This is probably the cause of fractures and breaks in the elderly. We know that peak bone mass is reached somewhere between the ages of 30 and 40. After this time, bone loss begins to occur at the rate of 0.3% per year.[4] There may be several reasons for this as we get older such as decline in physical activity, decline in muscle mass, and a lack of demands made upon the skeleton.

To prevent bone loss physical activity and exercise are necessary. This also will slow down the aging process. Taking calcium tablets with vitamin D are most beneficial in the prevention of this problem.

As we get older we see great changes in sleep variation. The amount of time spent in bed, total sleep and the number of awakenings all change as we get older. Older people spend more time napping during the day than younger people. Usually as we age less sleep is required. Even the quality of sleep changes due to various breathing problems which sometimes accompany aging.

The skin, the largest organ of the body, starts to become wrinkled. The complexion also changes in many older people. Muscle mass becomes less noticeable and fat deposits are more obvious. Then

---

3  Ibid., 114.

4  Ibid., 114.

there is the problem of losing teeth. It is so very important to visit a good dentist at least twice a year.

There are other signs of aging such as hearing loss due to a progressive bilateral loss of hearing (presbycusis) for tones and speech due to changes in the auditory system.[5] There are signs of aging such as the weakening of the immune system, glucose tolerance, cardiovascular function, the autonomic nervous system and the list goes on. The good thing about all of this is that we can slow down the process if we really want to.

We actually can slow down the aging process. Our bodies are composed of billions of cells each one requiring energy. The energy we use during the course of the day is brought about by the metabolic process which is the individual reactions of each cell. The cells in our bodies function for a time than they die and are replaced by new ones. Cells become old and are replaced by new ones but we don't understand how this process takes place the way that it does.

In cellular biology we realize that there are two important nucleic acids, namely, DNA, (deoxyribonucleic acid) and RNA (ribonucleic acid). The DNA tells the RNA how to build particular enzyme-proteins to carry out the functional intentions of each cell.[6] The quality of DNA will cause a good quality of RNA to be produced giving good energy to the cells causing peak perfor-

---

5 Dox, Melloni & Eisner, The Harper Collins Illustrated Medical Dictionary, 390.

6 Dhillon, Health, Happiness & Longevity, 116.

mance of each. If there is damage to the DNA it will be reflected in the poor function of the cells. If the cells become unable to divide and replace old cells, this will cause a defect in essential control systems or enzymes. Thus, aging will ensure. This has been an attempt to explain a most complicated process, but it will give us some idea of what is taking place.

Another theory that is prevalent about aging today is the free radical theory. This theory has long been associated with Vitamin E. Vitamin E is linked to energy and potency. Vitamin E is an antioxidant which alters the behavior of free radicals and oxidation reactions. We know that a free radical lacks an electron. For this reason they are most effective in damaging DNA and other cell structures. Free radicals can come about from the metabolic process or from contaminants in the environment. Foods that have been exposed to X-rays, cosmic rays and nuclear fallout will suffer free radical damage. This then is eaten by individuals which will cause damage to the DNA of the cells of the human body. Many believe that oxidation of a molecule causes it to become ineffective in its duties. So the free radical theory is based upon this explanation. Vitamin E., which is an antioxidant, will slow down oxidation and at the same time help slow down aging.

There are other theories about aging which we will not take into consideration at this time but we will look at things we can do to win the battle at least for a period of time. There are no miracles about slowing down the aging process but there are good things you can do to help yourself stay younger for a longer period of time.

There are some positive things that all of us can do to slow the aging process such as taking antioxidants. The free radical-oxidation theory of aging would support the idea of taking antioxidants to slow down the process of aging. Using Vitamin E to slow down aging has a great deal of support by scientists today who have studied the effects of Vitamin E on the heart and circulation. Vitamin C, which is also an antioxidant, has great potential for destroying free radicals in the body. Vitamin C will not totally destroy free radicals but will assist in their destruction, thus slowing down the aging process. Dr. Linus Pauling, Nobel Laureate in Chemistry and Peace, suggests that we use 2 grams of Vitamin C a day coupled with 1,200 units of Vitamin E.[7] There is only one problem that is, if we take too much of a good thing it can become an element in which cellular oxidation might be impaired.

Selenium has been known for a long time as an excellent antioxidant. Selenium is found in a wide variety of foods especially vegetables. Many American adults are low in selenium since the soil on which some of our foods are grown has become depleted of this important trace mineral. Especially in some of the Northern states, selenium is either very low in the soil or absent from it totally. Taking selenium, Vitamin C and Vitamin E may offer hope for all of us in slowing down the aging process.

---

7  Ibid., 118.

Another important thing all of us need to do is to limit the amount of polyunsaturated fat in our diet. Polyunsaturated fat is one of those substances that is oxidized quickly by the body and gives rise to more free radical damage. This will cause an increase in free radical damage to the cells. Polyunsaturated fat has been suggested for years to be used in place of butter and other fat spreads. It does help lower cholesterol but all dietary fat should be greatly reduced in the diet. Studies have shown that the use of polyunsaturated fats in the diet of rats has reduced their life span substantially.[8] The best thing that all of us can do is just not use polyunsaturated fats at all but to use a tiny bit of butter on our breads. Butter can be used by the body without the complications of other man-made spreads.

We need to consider the life-lengthening effects of dietary restriction as it helps promote a stronger immune system. There are times when the immune system fails to recognize its own cells and begins to attack them as foreign entities. Life can be prolonged if we use wisdom in eating only those things we know that will help our bodies. There are so many foods out there that just don't promote a good quality life and actually can be detrimental to long life.

Studies have shown that dietary restriction affects the immune system in a good way by slowing the harmful effect of attacking the body's own cells. Just by restricting our diets, by eating less, but eating the proper amounts of nutritious foods, will increase the

---

8   Ibid., 118.

life expectancy of the average individual. This work has been done by Dr. R. Walford of UCLA who also has shown that a lower body weight by twenty percent will add many years to the life of an individual. The benefits of lower weight reduces the chances of heart disease as well as diabetes.[9]

Some work has been done on the subject of nucleic acid damage because of age. Nucleic acids are found in such fish as sardines, kippers, salmon and other shell fish. It is believed that eating such a diet rich in nucleic acids will cause our cells to function as well as a younger individual. There is one problem with this diet in that it will create a lot of uric acid which can be damaging to the system. People with gout should not eat this diet unless they are prepared to drink gallons of water every day to prevent uric acid build up in the feet.

Foods that most vegetarians eat are very high in nucleic acids. Oily fish may cause adverse reactions and even raise cholesterol. Pinto beans and other beans, lentils, peas, asparagus, mushrooms and spinach are excellent sources of nucleic acids. Perhaps this may explain to some degree why vegetarians live longer than meat eaters and have less health problems.

As we conclude this chapter, we realize that good nutrition a diet high in fiber, very little meat in the diet and the exclusion of sugar from the diet will help prolong life. Vitamin E and C and foods rich in nucleic acids all contribute to a healthier and longer life.

---

9  Ibid., 119.

Exercise is most important in the pursuit of longevity. Exercising three to four times a week will keep the body in good condition and muscle tone and bone mass will be maintained more readily. More will be spoken about exercise in another chapter.

Eating To Win Beyond 2000 A.D.

# CHAPTER EIGHT

# THE MOST IMPORTANT DISCOVERY OF OUR AGE: FASTING

Have you ever thought about what you would consider the most important discovery of our age? In my opinion, it's got to be fasting. Today as never before we need to consider the need of fasting as a permanent part of our life style. Man holds within himself the very key to longevity. With the proper understanding of fasting and actually doing it, we can create within ourselves the quality of agelessness. At last we have come to understand that "fasting" is the greatest discovery of our time since its benefits are utterly amazing. Studies have shown an improvement in health of those who fast on a weekly basis.

Fasting has been used for thousands of years as a means of spiritual attainment and discipline. It is a way of purifying and cleansing the body. Those programs which limit food intake to teas, juices and broths are also considered fasts.

Europeans for the past two centuries have had spas in Switzerland, Germany and Austria where fasting was conducted under the supervision of the medical profession. During those times it was not uncommon to fast as long as 30 or even 40 days just on water.

Fasting in America has never been comprehended to the degree that Europeans have been enlightened to this ancient practice. We now know that our foods are contaminated by the way in which our farmers have used pesticides, insecticides, fungicides and other harmful chemicals. With the problem of air and water pollution these chemicals tend to remain within the human body. Fasting on juices or broths will help eliminate them in a slow manner from the body. Unfortunately, water fasts today have the tendency to cause unwanted symptoms such as diarrhea and nausea. This is the result of releasing toxicity too quickly from the body. It is best to use juices and broths for a period of time until the habit of fasting is well established as a part of a life style.

The problem of modern day farming is that it uses so many deadly chemicals against insects and plant diseases. These insecticides become a part of the plant as it grows. We can wash away those that are found on the surface of our vegetables but those that remain within the plant cannot be destroyed even during cooking.

Fasting is a wonderful way of getting rid of those toxins from the body. It must be understood that fasting should be exercised with caution and wisdom. Fasting helps to flush those poisons out of the body.

Our medical professionals are warning us of the danger of eating apples, pears, plums, green peppers and cucumbers because they have been coated with a solution of paraffin wax. This cannot be broken down by the liver and it presents one of the great health problems in America today.

The coating on the fruits and vegetables seals the products with a protective layer which retains the water and juices. It certainly retains the beauty of the product but it raises havoc with the human body. There isn't any organ in the human body capable of handling this deadly preservative. You will see the build up of wax on an apple when you put it under the hot water faucet as the wax slowly turns white and loosens its hold from the apple. When we come home from the grocery story, we put all the apples in a sink full of water and add a drop or two of bleach to cleanse them from what man has put upon them. All the fruit should be washed in this manner.

This wax must not remain in our bodies so a fast of twenty-four hours to thirty-six hours once a week should dispel this unwanted chemical from our bodies.[1]

Traditional fasting is combined with steam baths, special showers, breathing exercises and various

---

1  Paul C. Bragg, N.D., Ph.D. <u>Miracle of Fasting</u>,(Health Science, Santa Barbara, CA., 1981),26.

herbal teas and broths. During our fasting time let us use wisdom by drinking more than enough liquids to flush out the poisons from our bodies.

With the use of common table salt in America as a part of seasoning in our diets, we need to know how destructive this chemical can be to our bodies. Salt is not a food product. There is no reason why it should be used at all in our diet.

Salt cannot be digested, assimilated, or even used by the body. Salt does not contain any vitamins or trace minerals. It has absolutely no nutritional value whatsoever. Salt is harmful and may actually bring on problems in the kidneys, bladder, heart, arteries and blood vessels. It has the tendency to cause tissues to retain unwanted fluids in the body.[2]

Salt irritates the lining of the digestive tract and can rob the body of needed calcium. Salt is a habit we just don't need in our lives. There has been a misconception that salt is needed by the body. This is just not so. There are cultures of people throughout the world who have never tasted it. Once the salt habit is gone digestion improves.

While ministering in a Church in Memphis, Tennessee, we met a lovely lady who came forward for prayer. Rev. O. S. was nearly deaf because for 29 years she sprayed her sinus cavities with saline solution which contains salt. This resulted in a sodium overload in her body causing deafness and she had to leave the

2  Dr. N. W. Walker, D.Sc., <u>Health, Happiness, and Longevity</u>, (O'Sullivan Woodside & Company, Phoenix, Arizona, 1984), 44.

ministry because she could not hear what was being said to her. We advised her to stop this treatment immediately and we prayed for her. The Lord was merciful and His Healing power touched her and healed her of this deafness.

We know that salt for African Americans is a major contributor to hypertension and other unwanted diseases. Data indicates that African Americans are great users of salt as part of their daily dietary regiment.

Only by fasting can we turn around the possible damage that salt may be doing to your body. A twenty-four hour to thirty-six hour fast will help you eliminate the sodium build-up in your body. Not only will the salt begin to leave but other poisons and toxins will be flushed out.

We either rejuvenate ourselves or destroy ourselves by our wrong habits of living. If poisons are not from our bodies they will find a place to cause pain and damage. It is so important to build ourselves up by fasting. Fasting removes the toxins in a natural manner thus allowing the body to experience renewed energy. Aches and pains which might have bothered us in the past begin to slowly disappear. The toxins which found their way into the skeletal area between our joints will be released from the joints. It will take time but there will come improvement.

Fasting is a means by which Nature can unlock her store houses of energy that lies within our bodies.[3] The

---

3  Bragg, <u>Miracle of Fasting</u>, 22.

glorious thing about fasting is that it reaches every organ of the body. The body begins its internal house cleaning and you will be utterly amazed after you finish your fast to have renewed strength and energy.

The animal kingdom knows instinctively about fasting. When an animal in the wilderness becomes sick, it stops eating and goes on a natural fast to cure itself. This is the only means by which an animal has in finding a cure for itself. God put this wonderful instinct in them and they use it whenever necessary. Shouldn't we who have a higher intelligence practice fasting on a regular basis?

Autointoxication is an enemy against health and longevity.[4] Yet so many good people do not know that they are filled with toxins and poisons. Many times our moods are determined by this dreadful state found within the body. Worry, tension and anxiety are unnatural to healthy blood flow. The blood becomes loaded because we have not taken the time to fast and do internal house cleaning. Often times our negative state of mind can be attributed to autointoxication and an unclean blood supply. The Word of God presents us with an encouraging thought in I Peter 5:7, "Cast all your care upon him; for he careth for you." Surely our Heavenly Father will help us unload the worries and anxieties of daily living which will enhance a positive state of mind and grant us a healthy blood flow. The worse thing about autointoxication is that it is a state of the body which has taken years to come about. Only

---

4  Ibid., 26.

fasting can reverse this dreadful condition. Fasting coupled with natural eating will improve the entire state of the body. You will be utterly shocked to find out how good you begin to feel when you have fasted on a regular basis over as period of time. Each person is different and results will always vary but the benefits for all are certainly worth the effort.

Autointoxication is an enemy to the existence of your very life. It is the root cause of every major disease that might assail you and it exists in the blood because we have not done internal cleansing. Our poisoned blood stream has more to do with aging than any other cause known to mankind. Fasting will assist in removing the poisons from our blood and ensure a longer life span.

Dr. Paul Bragg, an outstanding naturopathic physician, would tell his listeners that a person with a sound constitution according to natural science should easily live until 120 years of age. If we will eat correctly, exercise, drink pure water and fast weekly, old age will be a blessing and not a curse.

For thousands of years people of all cultures have known about the benefits of fasting. Now let us take a look at some of them.

1) Fasting cleanses the body of toxins and poisons.

2) Fasting will speed up the detoxification process.

3) Fasting will stimulate the bowels and aid in eliminating impacted feces.

4) Fasting helps in restoring the cells and tissues to a more youthful condition.

5) Fasting assists the body in releasing its rejuvenating powers.

6) Fasting will enhance our energy levels.

7) Fasting aids in regulating body function.

8) Fasting promotes both spiritual and soulical peace.

9) Fasting will cause our mental faculties to become more alert.

10) Over a period of time fasting will aid in normalizing blood pressure.

These are just a few of the marvelous benefits of fasting. There are so many more that you will experience when you decide to make fasting a part of your life.

Before one really chooses to fast they need to take a good look at themselves both physically and spiritually. If you are suffering from low blood pressure, cancer, diabetes, heart disease, gout, liver or kidney disease or if you are taking prescribed drugs for any health condition, see your doctor first. It is important that you fast but at the same time there are some people who must not fast and you may be one of them. See your doctor if any physical or mental problems exist at this time.

There are those people who fast one day a week and do very well with it. There are others who need to know how to fast and how to prepare themselves for a fast. If you are going to fast for a day at a time once a week, than about two days before your fast start eating vegetables and fruits and totally cut out meat for those days. Make sure during your fast you drink pure steamed distilled water and fresh juices cut in half with this water. Do not just fast alone on steam distilled water because you may have reactions if you're only doing a water fast. Drink at least a quart of juice during your fast but remember to cut this in half with water. This will prevent pancreatic shock. Drinking juices alone is not advisable since the body could go into sugar shock. Drink as much water as you like on a fast.

A word of caution: never fast without drinking water. There are those who fast three days at a time without taking in liquids. They believe that this is God telling them to do so. If that is the case, how do you explain the kidney damage which occurs on such a fast? Always drink water on your fast and juice cut in half with water.

If you're planning to fast for an extended period of time, please prepare yourself with a few smaller fasts several weeks before you launch out on a prolonged fast. Use wisdom and the blessing of the fast will be apparent.

In the early stages of a fast you may experience acidosis of the blood, low blood sugar, headache, depression, fatigue or the very opposite of this which is hyperactivity. Never fast beyond three days unless you are under the supervision of an expert in the area of fasting.

Do not drink coffee or black tea during your fast. Your stomach will certainly tell about the foolishness of this act. During the course of a three day fast there will be no nutritional loss. If an individual fasts beyond reason, they will do terrible damage to their body. The body will begin to burn its own protein. This is called catabolism. It is so necessary to heed these warnings or your fast will be a nightmare and not a blessing.

Try to drink at least two quarts of water every day during your time of fasting. The liquids from boiled potatoes, garlic, celery and carrots are excellent sources to combat acidosis (high acidity) during your fast. Cut up the potatoes (skins left on), fresh garlic, celery and carrots and place them in a deep pot filled with water and boil for about 20 to 30 minutes. Let this mixture cool and drink it during the fast. It will help counteract the acidity which might occur. If you are on a twenty-four hour fast the vegetables may be eaten when the fast has come to an end. You must not break the fast with these since the stomach will not be prepared for such a large amount of food. A small tossed salad with a glass of juice (cut in half with water) is the only way to start eating again after a short fast.

If you have been on a three day fast, start with a small portion of an orange or grapefruit and drink only a small amount of distilled water. It is very important to chew the fruit very slowly to prevent your digestive system from getting over taxed.

On the second day of breaking a long fast, try eating cooked (steamed) brown rice or a baked potato and a small garden salad.[5] On the third day after a prolonged fast, again try a baked potato and a small garden salad. The fourth day eat only a vegetarian meal. More than one meal is permissible if your stomach is able to cope with the food.

Fasting is not a cure all but it certainly can change conditions in the body for the better if practiced on a regular basis. A regimen of fasting combined with juicing will work wonders for those who are seeking renewed strength and energy. Fasting has the propensity of revitalizing the body and giving it a sense of youthfulness. Try this program for several months and see if you are not more healthy. You will have a feeling of joyful youthfulness.

During your fast try using teas such as peppermint, chamomile and rose hips. These three teas have been known to have healing properties. It has been known that chamomile is a relaxant and most wonderful just before bed. Rose hips has been used in England over the centuries for detoxifying the body during the fast. It is very high in Vitamin C. Peppermint tea has been known to help restore the good bodily functions.

Remember to drink at least 2 quarts of steam distilled water each day while on a prolonged fast. Your daily liquid intake will be about 2½ quarts of all liquids combined together. Try having two good showers a day during the fast to eliminate the odor

---

5  Ibid., 65.

that will be apparent from your body. Use castile soap as it restores the balanced ph of the skin, is natural and most beneficial for the entire body. Have you ever tried washing your hair in this soap?

During the course of your fast, mild exercise is commendable. Walking is perhaps the best activity that can be done for most of us while fasting. Those living in the "deep freeze" of Northern America will have to choose another type of exercise during the winter as the climate may be unsuitable for outside activities. If you are used to vigorous exercise, be most cautious of doing this during a prolonged fast.

There is an aspect of fasting which we must consider in this chapter. As we get older, it would seem that we loose the elasticity and resiliency in our bodies. This does not necessarily have to come about. Between our joints we have what is called synovial fluid.[6] This fluid allows us to move freely and without pain. If this fluid becomes polluted with uric acid crystals the joints will become stiff and in some cases even cemented.

Just because we are getting older, this does not mean that we should loose our freedom of movement. There should be no diminishing of the supply of synovial fluid to the joints of our body.

Because we have been accustomed to eating incorrectly through the years, toxic crystals will begin to form within the body. Toxic crystal build-up takes years before it appears between the joints. These toxic

---

6  Ibid., 33.

acid crystals attack the moveable joints and attach themselves on the joints and calcified substances replace the synovial fluid. The joints which are attacked become painful and in some cases begin to swell.[7]

The attack on the joints usually begins in the extremities of the feet and hands. The feet are highly susceptible to this since there are 26 movable bones in the feet. The feet have more movable joints than other parts of the skeleton. Another reason for this is that gravity draws the toxic crystals to the feet. Lubrication between the moveable joints in the feet and hands becomes less and less.[8]

The acid crystals do not stop just with the feet and hands. If the toxicity is not dealt with by fasting on a regular basis, it will begin to attack the lower back and spine. Spurs will form. Again please understand that fasting is not a cure, but it will certainly bring relief. Since these acid crystals that are in the body are poisonousness they will attack the movable joints of the body.

We all need to fast for the purification of the body. When we fast for twenty-four hours or thirty-six hours, the healing power of the body begins to be released. Since the body is becoming cleaner on a regular fasting schedule, the over-all health of the individual will improve. Please understand that it is

---

7  Ibid., 37.

8  Ibid., 37.

going to take time to break down these toxic crystals in the body. It took years to bring them about and now it is going to take time for them to be eliminated from the system. To the degree that one is toxic will be the degree of time needed for fasting to do its job.

Every time we fast, we will notice more freedom in all of the movable joints of our bodies. A sense of agelessness will replace that tight, stiff aching feeling.[9] As you add natural foods to your diet not only will you feet better but you will look younger.

The Bible gives 74 references to fasting and is full of examples of men and women who fasted frequently. Moses, Elijah and David knew the tremendous value of fasting. We realize that Jesus received great power after His forty day fast in the wilderness. Moses fasted forty days and came down from the mountain only to go back to the mountain and fast another forty days. Moses fasted without drinking water. This is something that you must never do! Moses was called by God to fast and his fast was a supernatural one. We just need to fast! Very few are ever called by the Lord to do such fasting as Moses did.

There are those today who will tell you that you should never fast. They are ignorant of the value and benefits of fasting. They believe that it is unscientific and that you might do permanent damage to your body. They just don't know how glorious it can be. Many will tell you that you must eat in order to have

---

9 Dr. N. W. Walker, D. Sc., <u>Become Younger</u>, (O'Sullivan Woodside & Company, Phoenix, Arizona, 1984), 183.

your strength. This is just not so. On a long fast you definitely feel poorly for the first few days but after that your energy will increase. You will lose your appetite and food cravings will become less and less as your fast continues. Remember you're loaded with toxic waste and as your body flushes out these poisons you probably will feel some discomfort. There is only a slight unpleasantness but the benefits will out weigh the momentary affliction.

Just this past week I heard a man tell me at one of my seminars how he must eat three times a day or he just can't handle life. He told all of us that he eats whether he is hungry or not. He is now about sixty pounds over weight and has an impacted colon. He suffers from regular constipation and takes laxatives for his difficulties. He has no conception of the health benefits of fasting nor will he even try. He had become a "food-o-holic". Being totally addicted to food and never seeing a way out of this hidden dilemma is so typical of countless Americans. When we fast we give our digestive systems a most needed rest. Consequently the entire body will become enervated.

Fasting has been a true blessing to so many people because after the fast the stomach shrinks. This then will allow the over-weight individual to eat less with the consequences of losing extra pounds.

If you want all the benefits of fasting you must take a step and plan your fasting schedule today. Be rigid about this and don't let anyone or anything get in your way of fasting unless the Lord dictates otherwise.

As you plan your fasting schedule keep this strictly confidential. In this manner you will avoid the remarks and questions of those around you who do not have the insight into God's miracle plan of detoxification. Your body will respond with renewed energy, vigor and strength. Your skin will take on a new glorious tone. Your eyes will sparkle but above all your internal organs will feel most youthful. Much poison will leave your body and you will certainly notice the difference.

Yes, there will be light headedness and perhaps a little diarrhea on the fast. This is normal and it should not alarm you. This is your body telling you that poison is leaving. If you're taking medications, please consult with your doctor before you do any fasting. Again people with chronic disease must consult their physician before any attempt is made at fasting.

If you have truly made up your mind to fast, try fasting for a day by going on a twenty-four hour fast. During this time you will eat nothing but you will drink water (steam distilled water) for twenty-four hours. You may drink juice provided that it is cut in half with water. You must not take your routine and mineral supplements or your fiberblend while on a one-day fast since you will eat no food. This is going to be a life-style change for you which will only bring improvements to your over all health.

If you experience a headache on your fast, this is due to the fact that the coffee habit, the tea habit or the alcohol habit (stimulate habit) is being dealt with by the body trying to expel some of the poison that comes from these habits.

During your twenty-four hour fast you should be able to carry on your normal duties without interruption. There may be a little turbulence in the stomach but do not be alarmed. Remember you are in charge of telling your body what to do.

The more often you have a twenty-four hour fast during the course of the year, the easier it will become for you to fast for longer periods of time. Your weekly fast will help with internal house cleaning. A longer fast will definitely help in cleaning out the wastes and poisons which have accumulated during the course of your life. Do not attempt a long fast until you have mastered the 24 hour fast and the 72 hour fast. If you wish to do a longer fast, please find someone who has knowledge of fasting so that your fast will be supervised.

So we can say in conclusion that fasting is God's way of keeping His children healthy and strong. All of us need to practice fasting as a way of preventing disease. Naturally for many of us fasting may be rather difficult since we like our food so very much. With time and effort we can over-come those negative aspects of our thinking about fasting when we see and feel the great results this ancient practice brings.

Eating To Win Beyond 2000 A.D.

# CHAPTER NINE

# EXERCISING TO MAINTAIN MAXIMUM HEALTH

It is not possible to over emphasize the importance of consistent exercise if you want to be healthy and maintain the blessing of your life style change.

Whatever might have troubled you before, there is a good way to deal with the numerous physical complaints that you might have experienced. Nothing can help or cure faster than a good brisk walk. It cannot cure everything but walking causes the circulation to speed up the heart. It will take off the edge of nervous tension. It aids in relieving anxiety and daily frustration. The rewards that walking offers equal those of such outstanding sports such as swimming and even snow skiing. Walking helps maintain your weight and even aids in taking weight off. It helps in keeping bones from being weakened and even improves your looks. It gives the individual an opportunity to think and pray, if they so desire. Walking in the evening aids in relaxation and sleep becomes improved.

Walking causes more oxygen to be taken into the bloodstream. This will assist in recovery from illness and accidents. We know that blood pressure is lowered and gout is prevented by causing increased frequent urination. This will lower the uric acid level which is responsible for gout. The body becomes more flexible and arteries more elastic. Walking is a most wonderful way of improving over-all health.

If walking is combined with a natural diet (vegetarian) this will be a defense against the aging process. Diet and exercise help prevent atherosclerosis and the tragic results of that disease. Remember that walking helps stimulate the intestines to function more quickly. Walking with diet will help lower cholesterol.

If you have not been a walker it is best that you start out slowly. It would even be advisable to consult your doctor before starting a walking program. Start with a short distance in which you will be comfortable. Take three to five days before you increase your distance. After a good week of walking try to double your distance. If you increase your distance about 10% every three to four days you will have double your distance in a very short time.[1]

It is not important in the beginning how fast you're walking. The speed will increase as your body

---

1  Sukhraj S. Dhillon, Ph.D., <u>Health, Happiness, & Longevity</u>, (Japan Publications, Inc., New York, New York, 1983), 140.

becomes conditioned to walking. This will probably take about five weeks. If you're able to walk four or five miles in about five weeks time then you might try jogging.

Always be careful about your speed whether your walking or jogging. Checking your heart rate is the best indication of your physical condition. If your pulse is 100 after walking or jogging for a minute than things appear to be just fine. If your pulse exceeds the 130 count, do less walking or jogging. When you're in shape your pulse should be around 100 per minute. It is so very important to do this because you do not want to exceed your present level of activity until your heart is conditioned.[2]

As we are learning to eat to win, at the same time we must not make excuses for not exercising. Try walking either in the morning before you have to be at your place of employment. If this is not possible try walking after your evening meal. It will help with the digestion and give you time to think about what is really important in your life.

Make a walking schedule so that you will maintain a daily habit of this wonderful exercise. It is not always possible in the winter to walk out of doors but you sure can try your local mall. Some malls across the country encourage senior citizens to walk in the mall by marking down a starting point and a finishing point. The walkers are able to measure the miles they walk indoors at the malls where the owners encourage

2  Ibid., 140.

exercise. Make walking a part of your life. Remember you only go around once and your health is vitally important. Ask your wife or husband or a good friend to walk with you and the both of you will benefit greatly.

Try parking your car a short distance from your place of employment and walk the rest of the way. Don't take an elevator but try walking up the stairs for a change. This will strengthen your heart and increase your breathing capacity.

Always walk naturally and with a brisk pace while taking your walk. The average individual should be able to do about 120 steps after a good month of walking.

Don't make excuses for not exercising. Your health is at stake. You can prevent a heart attack and even premature death by exercising at least four to five times a week.

There are those who prefer a more strenuous exercise so they may desire to be involved in sports such as baseball, football or basketball. Such folks like to be involved in these activities for various reasons. Those of us who have less time need to be involved in "aerobics".

All aerobic teachers will tell you that your exercise program should include stretching and strengthening exercises. While doing your aerobic exercises you burn calories at a very fast rate. This is partially due to the metabolism speeding up by as much as ten percent.[3]

If you have a weight problem, be encouraged that aerobics burns more calories for heavy people than for thin individuals. At the same time you will see your energy levels increased with better concentration and a sounder sleep.[4]

If weight loss is your goal, then aerobics are probably the best thing for you to do. Dancing, swimming, vigorous walking, cycling, roller skating, biking, running, power walking and cross country skiing are excellent aerobic exercises. These burn fat at a faster rate because more energy is needed to do the exercise itself.

Many people benefit greatly from strength building exercises. You can even do strength building exercises while at the same time doing some of your aerobic workout. Most strength building programs are based on the use of free standing weights. Bar bells and dumb bells are used most for strengthening programs but at the same time there are specialized machines you can use. At fitness centers you will find such machines as Universal, Cybex and Nautilus. These are not inexpensive machines and must be used under the supervision of a good instructor.

Body building requires discipline and great attention to detail while the body is being sculptured. It takes

---

3  Carlson Wade, <u>Nutritional Healers</u>, (Parker Publishing Company, Inc., West Nyack, N.Y., 1987), 152.

4  Ibid., 152.

time and great effort, but again the rewards are worth the effort and money.

Another most excellent exercise is jumping rope. Please know that jumping rope is not just for kids. It is a most cost efficient exercise. Agility, improved reflexes, toning your waist, hips, and legs are the great results of being faithful to a jump rope exercise.[5]

Buy yourself a good sturdy leather rope with wooden handles and find a good hard surface on which to jump. Jump for three minutes, rest one minute, then jump for another three minutes. This is more difficult then you can imagine. It is going to take some time before you can reach this level of exercise. If you count your warm-up exercises and cool-down time, you're going to have a seven to ten minute fabulous aerobic workout.

Remember to keep your arms straightened at your sides, and swing the rope over your head using an easy wrist motion. Make sure your knees are slightly flexed and put a light spring in your toes. You can do all kinds of variations with the rope as you become skilled at this exercise.

There are so many good opportunities these days to find a good gym where you can have a personal trainer to assist you. Remember it is your health and if you don't do something about your health, nobody else will.

---

5 Michael Oppenheim, M.D., The Man's Health Book, (Prentice-Hall Inc., Englewood Cliffs, N.J., 1994), 54.

One of the most important things you must do while walking is to have a good pair of shoes. Make sure your shoes fit well and are comfortable. Wear cotton or wool socks since they will absorb perspiration.

Bodily exercise is required of us all, whether living in the city or in the country, to promote health and strength. Regular exercise will benefit the entire spirit, soul and body; walking is one of the best cures of all.

My sister-in-law has acquired the habit of walking every evening after the supper dishes are done. She and her youngest son walk out on the side of the farm road near their home in the cool of the evening. The day is behind them and there is peace as they see it come to a close. The Wisconsin winter does not hinder their walk because they know how to dress and enjoy the crisp, crackling snow under them. It is their time to share and relate as a mother to her son, at the same time prepare themselves for a restful night's sleep. Would that each of us could enjoy such luxury of undisturbed exercise while enriching the soul and the spirit.

Eating To Win Beyond 2000 A.D.

## CHAPTER TEN

# FOR MEN ONLY: YOU'RE NOT A KID ANY LONGER

Every year in the United States about 40,000 men will die of prostate cancer. This terrible disease is on the increase among the men of this country. Most men don't know what the function of the prostate is and where it is located.

If you are a man somewhere over the age of fifty, you need to know about your prostate gland. Have you been having frequent urination, especially at night? This problem may not be with your bladder but with your prostate gland. Especially if you're making frequent trips to the bathroom at night, this could be a disorder of your prostate.

This walnut-sized organ called the prostate is located next to the bladder. It is in the bladder that the urine is stored. The prostate surrounds the urethra. The urethra is the canal through which the urine passes out of the body. The prostate gland produces the liquid that acts as a vehicle for the sperm cells which, during intercourse, are secreted into the vagina. The purpose of this is the fertilization of the female's egg. The end of this is the normal process of reproduction. Without this wonderful little gland, the male will become sterile.

A normal walnut-sized prostate gland appears like a small bunch of grape-like bulbs, wrapping itself around the urethra and it empties it's fluid into that tube at the moment of orgasm. When the prostate is abnormal in size, it puts pressure on the urethra, thus increases the time to empty the bladder. As the prostate enlarges, the greater the pressure and the more difficult it becomes to totally empty the bladder.[1]

If you are having a hard time with your prostate gland here are a few warning signs.

With prostatitis there is always a feeling of congestion and discomfort in the pubic area.[2] The bladder always feels as though it is full, with the necessity of making frequent trips to the bathroom especially during the night hours. On occasions it will become most difficult to void; rarely there will be no passage of urine at all.

The need to urinate during the night hours is most distressing. It interrupts your sleep. Then there is the problem of waste residue collecting in the bladder, but some release may be possible. This condition can become serious if the urethra becomes blocked. The

---

1   Carlson Wade, <u>Nutritional Healers</u>, (Parker Publishing Company, Inc., West Nyack, N.Y., 1987), 181.

2   Ibid., 182.

probability of uremic poisoning arises when the bladder becomes overloaded with fluid.[3] If the waste is not discharged it can flood the kidneys, presenting a most serious danger of poisoning to the entire system.

Understand that prostate problems do not just go away and it is most advisable to see a physician as soon as possible. There is the possibility that the ailing prostate will become so enlarged it will constrict the urethra and completely block the flow of urine. This condition is extremely painful and could be fatal if not treated at once.

Here is a list of warning signals that might indicate problems with the prostate.

1) Pain in the lower back.

2) The presence of blood in the urine or in the seminal excretion.

3) Frequent erections without any prior stimulation.

4) Pain during the release of the seminal fluid.

5) Failure in erection (impotence and/or premature ejaculation).

6) A persistent sense of fullness in the bowels and difficult in elimination of waste.

7) Difficulties either in starting your stream or the inability to stop the flow of urine could mean a loss of control over urination.

---

3  Ibid., 182.

Men over fifty years of age should have their prostate gland checked at least once a year. This is a precaution which could assist in the prevention of serious health problems.

## Common Prostate Problems

Acute prostatitis is an inflammation of the prostate coupled with a bacterial infection.[4] The symptoms may include fever, chills and painful urination with possible pain in the lower back and between the legs.

Chronic prostatis is an infection which comes and goes. Symptoms of this disease are the same as the acute form but may be milder. Massaging the prostate has proven beneficial in releasing the blocked fluids.

Benign prostatic hypertrophy (BPH) is an enlargement of the prostate gland. This disease is related to small noncancerous tumors that grow inside the prostate.[5]

Prostate cancer is a malignant growth arising in the outer zone of the prostate. Today this disease claims one-third of the newly diagnosed cancers among men in this country. If the disease is not diagnosed early it may spread to other organs and death will occur. When symptoms do appear they are similar to those of BPH. BPH is related to the changing hormone level as one ages.

---

4   The Harper Collins Illustrated Medical Dictionary, 1993 ed. s.v. "Prostatitis".

5   Encyclopedia Of Medicine, 1989 ed., s.v."Prostatitis."

A urologist is recommended to treat this disease. Since he is a specialist in disorders of the urinary system, his understanding of this disease has been greatly enhanced by special training.

The best way to protect yourself against this disease of the prostate is to have a yearly examination as previously mentioned. If symptoms occur go to your health care practitioner as soon as possible. It could save your life.

**Therapy**

Paramount to dealing with the disease of the prostate and prevention is an adequate intake and absorption of the mineral zinc. Studies show that zinc has actually reduced the size of the prostate. Zinc is probably so successful in the treatment of this disease of the prostate because it is involved with many aspects of hormonal metabolism.

The prostate accumulates very high levels of zinc, perhaps more than any other organ of the body. When benign hypertrophy is existent there is a deficiency of zinc.[6] This mineral is necessary for sperm function, sexual health and other reproductive hormone systems.

The prostate gland has about ten times as much zinc than any other gland of the body. Zinc has a unique influence on the sperms ability to swim. The sperm must be tenacious enough to swim to the woman's

---

6  Carlson Wade, <u>Nutritional Healers</u>, 184.

fallopian tubes so penetration of the egg will take place for fertilization.

Zinc may be found in brewer's yeast, nuts, eggs, rice bran, onions, chicken, beans, peas, lentils, wheat germ, wheat bran, beef liver and gelatin. Be cautious about the amount of eggs, chicken and liver that you eat since these have lots of cholesterol. Try to find as many other sources of food as you can to get the zinc you need. Zinc is also available at health food stores and pharmacies. It is believed that thirty-five milligrams per day of zinc will build up resistance to prostate disorders and even relieve the symptoms it produces.

Zinc actually acts as a catalyst in many biological reactions to nourish and even rejuvenate the prostate. Amino acids and nutrients are brought together by the zinc to aid in the repair of the delicate tissues and tubules of the prostate to keep it in a youthful condition. Since zinc plays a role in carbohydrate metabolism, the energy source is build into the prostate to keep it alive, healthy and young.[7]

Certainly as a child you ate pumpkin seeds. These wonderful seeds are full of vitamins and minerals and are an excellent source of vegetable protein. These tasty seeds are a source of essential fatty acids, which the prostate readily absorbs as the very essence for its life.

Essential fatty acids are well known for preserving the health, virility and even the potency of the

---

7   Ibid., 185.

prostate.[8] These concentrated nutrients in pumpkin seeds work in conjunction with zinc to keep the delicate tubules, cells and tissues in smooth working order. These nutrients actually enter right into the prostatic fluid maintaining the vigor, strength and fitness of the gland. Linoleic acid, linolenic acid, and arachidonic acid help keep the heart healthy and make a positive difference to your prostate.

If you don't like eating pumpkin seeds than you are able to buy pumpkin seed capsules at the local health food store. Pumpkin seeds and oil work like a miracle drug in prostate rejuvenation. Sunflower seed oil, wheat germ oil, soybean oil and sesame seed oil are full of EFAs. Walnuts, Brazil nuts, pine nuts, peanuts, pecans and almonds help the prostate to remain healthy.

Let us not forget the great benefits that come from garlic. Garlic is a powerful store house of natural antibiotics that help insulate the prostate from infection and bacteria. According to Professor Gurwitch, a European electrobiologist, garlic releases an ultraviolet radiation called mitogenetic radiations.[9] These rays have the ability of stimulating cell growth and activity of the prostate. Garlic appears to have a natural antibiotic property that would shield the prostate against parasitic infection. Garlic has the ability to assist in repair and reconstruct weakened glandular tissues so that the organ will remain healthy.

---

8   Ibid., 186.

9   Ibid., 187.

Garlic is full of allicin which has the propensity to cleanse away decomposed bacteria. Garlic helps prevent prostate infection since it has the ability to destroy certain strains of bacteria. Garlic possesses a powerful penetrative force unlike many other herbs.[10] Dr. Gurwitch's research indicates that garlic is able to uproot and discharge infections and bacteria which allow the prostate to regenerate itself. Garlic is most important for this gland. Cut up a few cloves of garlic and put them in a salad with pumpkin seeds. Try a tablespoon of sesame seeds for your dressing and you will have a powerful tonic for the prostate.

Remember to purchase or grow your foods that promote prostate health. Raw pumpkin or sunflower seeds, cold-pressed vegetable oils, garlic and essential fatty acids all contribute to prostate health.

In addition to all of the above, don't forget to eat your green and yellow vegetables. Studies have shown that men who eat these on a daily basis have a much lower rate of prostate cancer than those who don't eat these good foods.

Perhaps the key to all of this is that vegetables are high in Vitamin A and high in fibre. We talked about the need of colon cleansing in Chapter 7 and we stated that waste products from the bowels must be eliminated quickly. The fibre found in the vegetables pushes the waste through the intestines and colon very rapidly. This does not give the colon an opportunity for fermentation from the various negative bacteria.

10 Ibid., 188.

Cancer becomes less of a threat for the prostate and colon if the bowels are thoroughly cleansed.

It is time for all men to take good care of their prostate glands. Thousand of men die yearly since they fail to have an annual examination of their prostate. It is up to each man to take charge of his health care and to treat his prostate as he would any other organ of the body. You could prevent disease of the prostate by your own personal diligence. Take care of you whole body and enjoy God's blessing of a long life.

Eating To Win Beyond 2000 A.D.

# CHAPTER ELEVEN

# THE WAYS OF A WOMAN

God has fashioned women most uniquely with many mysterious elements that are difficult to understand. God said that she is "beautifully and wonderfully made". Yet, as the little girl enters her teen age years she will have years of menstruation ahead of her causing her to reconsider how "wonderfully" she really feels especially if premenstrual syndrome is one of the problems associated with those times of the month. Then as the lady enters into the mid-forties, she will have to adjust to another life-style change called the menopause. This chapter is written to help women cope with these twin problems by better nutrition and the adjustment needed during those times of her life.

There is a good nutritional approach to PMS (premenstrual syndrome) and menopause to aid women having these problems. Let us not forget that PMS is a real monthly hassle for many women. Men just don't have an understanding of what women actually go through each month. One major difference between a man's body and a woman's is that the women's hormones are in a continuous state of flux. A man's sex hormones remain more stable until they are needed to engage in the sexual act. When a woman is about to menstruate, she experiences both physical and emotional changes in her body. It is universally experienced by all women on planet earth. It is estimated that over 90 percent of women are said to have some form of premenstrual syndrome. The authorities do not all agree to what extent women in America suffer from this natural monthly occurrence. Some claim as much as 58 percent experience PMS; others say that only 3 to 15 percent have this experience. We know that as many as 10 percent will seek medical advice for this problem. Some women become frightened by sharp fluctuations in mood and depression swings. Others are shocked by the weight gain that accompanies the monthly cycle.[1] These hormonal changes are not grasped by many women which can cause unnecessary distress. The usual physical complaints are headache, bloating, fatigue and even insomnia.

Medical science believes that the causes of PMS are due largely to fluctuating hormonal irregularities during the monthly cycle. Often times symptoms will reoccur with regular predictions. As the cycle begins the ovaries produce the female hormone called estrogen. After ovulation, a second hormone, progesterone

---

1 Carlson Wade, <u>Nutritional Healers</u>, (Parker Publishing Company, Inc., West Wyack, N.Y., 1987), 191.

appears on the scene. Progesterone is needful for pregnancy, but it affects the lining of the uterus (endometrium) causing it to become thicker, and swelling accompanies this condition. In addition the general body tissues retain more sodium. Consequently, the sodium from salt draws more water and increases fluid build up. The space between the tissues swell and there is a weight gain. Other symptoms of PMS could be caused by swelling in the uterus, pelvis, abdomen, legs, liver and brain.[2] Some women cope very well with PMS but to others it is a living hell with much discomfort and emotional upheaval.

Confirmed medical research has shown that menstrual cramps are caused by a body chemical called prostaglandin.[3] The lining of the uterus contains this chemical but it is inhibited by the female hormone progesterone. This hormone is at peak levels about two weeks before the period begins. Its primary function is to help a nutrition-carrying blood supply reach the uterus on a monthly basis. The uterine wall blood build-up is God's way of preparation for pregnancy. When the brain receives information that the egg which has dropped is not fertilized, the progesterone level falls dramatically. Then the prostaglandin is released, so it can prompt the smooth muscles in the uterus to slowly return to normality. Thus the blood lining is pushed out.

---

2  Ibid., 192.

3  Ibid., 192.

If the body has a high level of prostaglandin, the uterus will contract rapidly bringing on pain, cramps and swelling. When prostaglandin spills over into the bloodstream, it will affect the smooth muscles (over which there is no conscious control). The smooth muscles include the muscles in the heart, blood vessels, intestines and naturally the uterus. Undoubtedly this is the reason so many women experience headache, backaches, nausea, diarrhea, dizziness, hot and cold flashes and cramping. If the prostaglandin should act up, they put the women on a hormonal roller coaster for ten days of each month. Some days the symptoms are mild but other days they can be severe. Is it any wonder that women feel frustration and despair? Blame this on the prostaglandins![4]

There are positive things you can do to help you through the monthly cycle. A change in diet and taking supplements will greatly reduce the symptoms of PMS.

Vitamin B6 or Pyridoxine is known to influence the release of neuro-transmitters (dopamine and serotonin) adding in stabilizing the fluctuating mood swings. Pain is eased with B6 causing the prostaglandins to be less devastating during the period. One of the good things about B6 is that it helps reduce bloating and speeds up the kidneys. It acts as a natural diuretic. Not only does this vitamin assist in relieving depression but it acts as an antispasmodic. Some good sources of B6 are brewer's yeast, potatoes, vegetables and deep water

---

4   Ibid., 193.

fish. Remember to take B6 with a good B complex vitamin since the B vitamins must work in conjunction with each other. Small doses of B6 are recommended such as five to ten milligrams and larger doses of this should be given under your physician's direction.

We live in an age when there are radio and television ads about the need of calcium and its benefits. It is so true especially with PMS since calcium levels in the blood drop substantially during the monthly cycle. When calcium is low this triggers such negative emotions as depression and nervousness. Some women complain of severe muscle cramps, edema and headaches. These are not imaginary symptoms but nagging complaints that calcium can alleviate. We know that calcium helps the heart beat normally and nerve conduction is improved but especially hormone secretions are better regulated when this mineral is present. Women taking calcium during menstruation do much better than others who do not take this supplement and about 1,000 to 1,500 milligrams daily will make a tremendous difference. Also, magnesium is needed to work in conjunction with calcium. Calcium breaks down better with magnesium but magnesium does not work well without B6. So you will also need B6 when taking this combination. Good sources of calcium may be found in cheese, Gruyere cheese, sardines and salmon. I do not recommend milk since adults do not need milk, which contributes to mucous build-up in the sinus cavities. Magnesium is found in nuts, soybean seeds, whole grains and green leafy vegetables.

If there is a deficiency of zinc in the body during PMS it could lower the body's resistance to infection and slow the healing process. There are emotional upheavals which are promoted during PMS such as headaches and nervousness which are linked to a zinc deficiency. It is best to take thirty to fifty milligrams of zinc per day during PMS. At the same time, the benefits of this mineral cannot be over estimated so it might be advisable to take zinc every day. Take it daily with food if there has been a known deficiency. Zinc is found in a variety of foods such meat, poultry, eggs, milk and whole grains.

During your monthly cycle make sure that you're eating food abundant in potassium since it helps regulate fluid retention. Good sources of potassium are bananas, oranges, sun-dried fruits and untoasted and unsalted nut meats.[5]

We all have heard about the benefits of taking Vitamin E for better heart function and circulation but little has been known about its ability to guard against fibrocystic breast conditions. It is believed that this vitamin helps avoid this condition. Vitamin E helps prevent oxidation of fatty substances such as Vitamin E, essential fatty acids and the adrenal, pituitary and sex hormones.[6] Vitamin E will help establish normal hormonal balance during PMS. Dosages should be around 400 to 800 units per day. Do not exceed this limit since it is known that Vitamin E can cause

---

5   Ibid., 194.

6   Ibid., 194.

tachycardia if dosages are as much as 1600 units per day. Don't abuse this wonderful vitamin.

Make sure during your monthly cycle that you get enough essential fatty acids. It is now believed that these acids help maintain the biological balance of the body. Two of the most important acids that are needed are linoleic and linolenic. These function as a blocking factor for other essential fatty acids. Good sources may be found in safflower, sunflower, corn, wheat germ, soybean and sesame seed oil. All you need is about two full teaspoons of any of these and you will meet your daily requirement. EFAs ( essential fatty acids) may be found in a variety of nuts such as Brazil nuts, pine nuts, peanuts, pecans and sunflower seeds.

There are some simple things you can do if you suffer from PMS. It doesn't cost anything except your personal effort to avoid certain foods.

As we have mentioned before in this book: Avoid Salt! It encourages water retention. Check very carefully what you buy in the supermarket because of the hidden salt (sodium) in certain products. Read the ingredients to see how much sodium is present in the food you select. Don't use salt from the shaker as it is pure poison.

During PMS don't use sugar of any kind because it acts as a triggering devise that causes eruption of endocrine responses known as PMS.[7] This will encourage a sugar upheaval which will make you feel

---

7  Ibid., 196.

like you're losing your composure. Basically cells will bind insulin and create a high sugar level thus creating a high blood sugar and PMS symptoms will set in.

It is most important that you avoid coffee during the time of PMS. Coffee causes the brain to be overstimulated and affects the central nervous system. It changes a woman's metabolic rate Coffee will create an internal situation whereby insulin increases, blood sugar drops and a low blood sugar level will ensue, thereby causing hypoglycemia.[8] It is best to avoid all products that contain caffeine such as tea, cola and chocolates. Be aware of buying over the counter products that contain caffeine. Be a wise, knowledgeable buyer and read the label before you take it to the check-out counter. Live out your day being caffeine-free and you will be happy that you did!

To be most comfortable during the time of your period, plan ahead. Get on a good nutritional program which has been described above. If you are under stress prior to your period, it is most essential to plan a good nutritional program which will help you immensely in reducing the symptoms described above. If you are having pain, try using a heating pad either on your lower back or over the area of your lower abdomen. The heat will help the uterus to relax and relieve cramping.

For a light muscle relaxer try using a combination of bananas with 6 ounces of skim milk, 1 tablespoon of wheat germ, 1 teaspoon nut meats and 1 teaspoon of

---

8  Ibid., 196.

brewer' yeast mixed in a blender for about four minutes. The minerals contained in this recipe will work with vitamins B6 and E to relieve contractions that are responsible for muscular pains and spasms.[9]

PMS is a biological fact of life and you, as a beautiful woman, do not have to accept the suffering of pre-menstrual syndrome. Use these nutritional insights to meet the challenges of the pain cycle and then really be the beautiful woman God made you to be.

## Menopause - A Natural Change

Like menstruation, menopause is experienced by all women on plant earth when they enter the Enlightened Age! Unfortunately, the ignorance regarding menopause is nearly as universal as the experience. When a woman becomes pregnant, she is taught everything about her pregnancy and is watched carefully, giving her much attention prior to the birth of a perfectly healthy baby. At the time of her labor, she is fully prepared for all that will be expected of her. But this is not so with menopause. Most women enter into the menopausal time of their life knowing nothing, perhaps not even knowing that they're are in it! Yet the sad part is that very little of this subject is talked about, and a sort of mysterious taboo exists around the subject. There is an appalling level of ignorance and denial about this change of life that is faced by half of the population of the world all the way back to prehistoric times.

---

9   Ibid., 198.

Menopause is that span of time during which the menstrual cycle wanes and gradually stops. It is commonly called the change of life and climacteric.[10] The word "menopause" is derived from the Greek "meno", meaning "month" and "pausis" which is literally translated "ending". It is during this period of time that the ovaries stop functioning and menstruation and child bearing cease.

Menopause is a natural physiologic process that results from the gradual aging of the ovaries. The ovaries are no longer able to perform the function of ovulation and estrogen production. Since estrogen production stops great changes take place within a woman's body. The uterine tubes shrink in size and become less capable of movement.[11] The uterus and the cavity of the uterus with the cervix decrease in size. With aging the vagina contracts and its' folds become shallower. The clitoris and external sexual organs become smaller in size; the breasts become less full and firm.

Menopause usually occurs sometime between the ages of 35 and 58. If it should occur before the age of 35, it is a premature menopause; after 58 it is called delayed menopause. Both premature menopause and delayed menopause could be indicative of a primary

---

10 <u>Encyclopedia and Dictionary of Medicine, Nursing, and Allied Health</u> 1983 ed., s.v. "Menopause".

11 Ibid., "Menopause".

endocrine disorder or gynecologic dysfunction. This should be evaluated by a gynecologist.[12]

The most frequent symptoms of menopause are hot flushes of the face, neck and upper body and excessive perspiration especially at night. Emotionally, the menopausal women suffers greatly from irritability, depression and anxiety which is probably related to psychologic factors as well as physiologic changes. It has been noted that women who keep themselves meaningfully active suffer less symptoms than those who don't keep themselves psychologically active.

There is no truth whatsoever that menopausal women are less attractive sexually or do not desire sex. As a matter of fact, most post menopausal women enjoy sex perhaps even more since there is no fear of getting pregnant.

A hot flash is the result of a rapid change in the diameter of the blood vessels which is termed as a vasomotor instability. A hot flash usually last about two minutes. It is best to dress in loose fitting clothing and remember, you can always remove a jacket or a coat. After the hot flash is over, you can always replace the jacket or the sweater.

Try to recall the kinds of foods that might trigger a hot flash. Don't smoke or drink any kind of alcohol and stay away from chocolate which just increases the intensity of the hot flashes. Keep your weight in control. Be aware that you don't take your problems

---

12 Ibid., "Menopause".

from work to your home with you. Get sufficient rest when needed. These simple little things will help you cope during those "Enlightened Years".

Eat a diet full of vegetables, whole grains, sea foods, legumes and low fat dairy products.

While going through the change, try to eat foods full of calcium and phosphorous. Spinach, milk, and spaghetti all contain these most essential trace minerals. Please do not cook the spinach or eat spinach from a can since cooked spinach creates a poison which can be harmful to the body.

If you will take good vitamins such as B-complex (found in whole grain foods), vitamin C (citrus fruits and juices) and Vitamin D (found in cod liver oil) these will assist in relieving the symptoms of menopause. Also try being out in the sun for a half hour a day for Vitamin D.

We can't underestimate the importance of Vitamin E in easing the symptoms of the menopausal woman. Vitamin E can be found in whole grains and vegetable oils. According to some physicians, people taking the heart medication digitalis should not take Vitamin E unless their physician says it is alright.

Again, exercise must be stressed in dealing with the symptoms of menopause. Walking, bicycling or swimming should be done at least four times a week to assist the body in maintaining bone integrity. Exercise helps avoid the dreaded disease of osteoporosis. Exercise helps your body to utilize calcium and other nutrients necessary for good health. Consult with your physician before starting an exercise program. You will be utterly amazed how much better you will feel with a weekly exercise program.

Menstrual difficulties are the result of hormonal upheaval that can be aided with nutritional therapy. By using these vitamin supplements such as Vitamin B6, calcium, zinc, potassium, Vitamin E and the essential fatty acids that are obtained from wholesome foods, you will lessen the symptoms and master this stage of life that is set before you.

You now have the knowledge of how to deal with this uniqueness. Women can gather up the rewards of moving through the Change of Life with peace and inner beauty and walk gracefully into their Golden Years that lie before them.

Eating To Win Beyond 2000 A.D.

## CHAPTER TWELVE

# CANCER AND NUTRITION

In 1993, more than 5 million Americans were diagnosed as having some kind of cancer. Currently, one out of every four Americans will develop some kind of cancer during his or her life time, and in that group of people at least one or more will die of that disease. It is estimated that one-third of all cancers are caused by cigarette smoking and other related tobacco habits. It is believed that 80 per cent of all cancers could be eliminated if people did not smoke or practiced other unhealthy habits.[1]

Cancer is not one disease but a group of diseases which affects the growth and duplication of healthy cells in the body. Normally, cells grow, divide and replace themselves in an appropriate manner. For some unknown reason which is not understood by scientists, cells begin to lose their ability to control their

---

1 James Marti and Andrea Hine, <u>Alternative Health Medicine Encyclopedia</u>, (Detroit, Michigan, Visible Ink Press, 1995), s.v. "Cancer".

growth, and begin to multiple in a haphazard manner. In the process, these abnormal cells can develop their own network of blood vessels that will siphon needed nourishment away from the body's blood supply.[2]

Every cell in the human body has the potential to turn cancerous. When the normal immune system is operating to capacity, it has the ability to destroy cancer cells or to reprogram them back to normal functioning. If the immune system becomes weakened or suppressed, it cannot destroy cancer cells neither is it able to reprogram them. Tumors begin to form which are masses of abnormal cells sometimes numbering in the billions before they become evident. If the cancer cells remain in one area, it is considered to be localized. Benign tumors usually are not life threatening. We see such tumors as warts and cysts and if they remain localized they can be removed by surgery.[3]

Malignant tumors are capable of developing in any organ of the body. These are composed of cells that multiply much faster than normal cells and have accompany abnormal chromosomes. Malignant cells are capable of traveling throughout the body. They enter the blood stream and migrate to the organs of the body. As they enter new organs they are capable of forming new tumors. Malignant tumors divert essential nutrients from these vital organs and release toxins into the blood stream and organ systems. They inter-

---

2 Ibid., Cancer.

3 Ibid., Cancer.

fere with the functioning of the organs so that serious illness and even death will ensure.[4]

Cancers are categorized according to the organ or type of tissue in which the tumor is located. There are more than 100 kinds of cancers. The five basic categories include carcinomas, sarcomas, myelomas, lymphomas and leukemias. Carcinomas are tumors that form in tissues that cover or line internal organs. Carcinomas account for about 80 to 90 percent of all known cancers. Intestines, lung, breast, prostate and skin are favorite sites for carcinomas.[5]

Sarcomas attack the connective tissues and muscles, cartilage and the lymph system. These types of cancers represent the smallest number of cancer cases, but are most likely to kill the patient. Bone marrow contains plasma cells which are attacked by myelomas. Cancer of the lymph glands or nodes are found in the neck, groin, arm pits and spleen and are known as lymphomas. The two most common lymphomas found in America are Hodgkin's disease and non-Hodgkin's lymphoma. Bone marrow, spleen and lymph nodes are favorite sites for tumors called leukemias. These are solid tumors which are characterized by excessive white blood cells.[6]

Most scientist do not agree on the causes of cancer. Most of them will agree that there is a common feature

---

4   Ibid., Cancer.

5   Ibid., Cancer.

6   Ibid., Cancer.

of all types of cancer and that is the rearrangement of the information found coded in the DNA within the single cells. There is a common consensus by our cancer scientists that environmental factors, including exposure to carcinogenic substances such as air pollution, tobacco smoke and industrial chemicals, are major factors to cancer. At the same time, diet, heredity, and lifestyle contribute in the development of cancer.

If we are to prevent cancer it is dependent upon each of us to avoid the risk factors linked with cancer. Our immune system must be maintained at peak performance to efficiently eliminate abnormal cells from the body. We are able to do this by adopting a diet that ensures the optimal intake of immuno-enhancing nutrients and decrease the intake of immuno-suppressing foods that weaken the immune system.[7]

We can avoid the cancer causing agents in our environment and eat the correct foods but at the same time if our mind and souls are not at peace we are at risk. Stress must be reduced and emotions muct be harmonious with our spirit. Our Lord Jesus tells us "Let not your heart be troubled, neither let it be afraid". His words are filled with peace and life and will aid in abating the cancerous growths.

There are several very good botanicals, herbs, which help in the prevention of cancer. Included in this list are spirulina, aloe vera, and green tea made from the leaves of camellia sinensis, echinacea, garlic, mistletoe,

---

7  Ibid., Cancer.

shiitake mushroom (extract of lentinus edodes), and maitake mushrooms.

Spirulina is a one-celled form of algae that multiplies in warm, alkaline fresh water bodies.[8] It is a Latin name derived from the word for helix or spiral because of it's form of swirling, microscopic strands.

Spirulina is known to have the highest source of Beta carotene, Vitamin B12 and gamma linolenic acid (GlA). Spirulina is a wonderful herb since it contains all nine essential amino acids that the body must derive from food intake.

Spirulina has many more times the Beta carotene than any other herb or vegetable including carrots. Spirulina is richer in B12 than liver as it contains 250 per cent more B12 and at least four times more protein than that of beef.

Spirulina contains 26 times more calcium than cow's milk. It also has lots of phosphorus and niacin. Spirulina is considered a complete food only with one exception and that it is lacking in carbohydrates. It is most beneficial for any and all aliments and if there has been a deficiency in the diet, the entire body will improve. Especially for those with cancer, this wonderful herb provides energy and improves strength. Spirulina is considered by herbalists to be one of Nature's whole foods.

---

8 Jack Ritchason, N.D., <u>The Little Herb Encyclopedia</u>, (3rd ed., Woodland Health Books, Pleasant Grove, UT. 1995), 244.

Aloe vera is one of the oldest therapeutic plants known by mankind. Aloes are a member of the plant group known as the Lily family. The term "Aloe" is from the Hebrew "halal", which means a shiming and bitter substance. "Vera" is from the Latin root "verus" which is translated as meaning "true".[9]

Aloe vera has been used by wholistic practitioners in the treatment of HIV which is related to the AIDS virus. It inhibits the virus from entering different cells and slows down the entrance to other cells. It stabilizes the individual's natural life force and contributes to balancing the blood.[10] It definitely boosts the blood which results in more energy for the patient. In the treatment of cancer we see a similar effect in boosting the immune system. It does balance the pH of the blood and helps with digestion and absorption. It is excellent in aiding the expulsion of toxins from the system. It helps promote the growth of friendly bacteria in the colon.

Cancer patients feel its effects almost from the onset of ingestion of the liquid or capsule. It is an energy booster and an immune enhancer.

Echinacea has been known by herbalists for centuries as the King of Blood Purifiers since it improves lymphatic filtration and drainage. In addition to this it has been found to help remove toxins from the blood. Some have even found it most beneficial in the

---

9  Ibid., 8.

10 Ibid., 10.

treatment of prostate problems since it causes the prostate to shrink to normal size.[11]

Echinacea is one of the most useful herbs available to Naturopathic Physicians since it has a wonderful ability to act as an antibiotic. It truly is a wonderful alternative to prescribed antibiotics. Echinacea is excellent in the treatment of vertigo and a confused mental state.[12]

Since echinacea is such a good blood cleanser by removing toxins, it is most beneficial in cancer therapy. It builds the immune system and helps the thymus gland to function by increasing its ability to create more killer T cells. Not only does it have antibiotic-like qualities but it acts also as a tumor suppressant.[13] Echinacea is most powerful against all kinds of bacterial and viral infections.

For hundreds of years people around the world have used garlic for their food but more especially as a natural medication against numerous diseases. Studies have shown that garlic can be used against infection of all kinds. It has been most successful for treating eyes, ears, nose and throat infections. The thiamin content in the herb is very high which helps build the immune system. Garlic contains a mineral called germanium which strengthens the immune system, and an antioxidant for aiding in physical endurance.[14] It has also been used in the treatment of wounds.

---

11 Ibid., 76.

12 Ibid., 76.

13 Ibid., 76.

14 Ibid., 92.

Garlic has also been shown to lower serum cholesterol and triglycerides. It has the propensity to raise HDL in healthy patients and helps those with coronary heart disease. It is known to protect the circulatory system against narrowing of the arteries. Studies have shown that garlic actually dissolves LDL, the harmful cholesterol, lowers triglyceride, and raises HDL, the good cholesterol.

These are just a few of the herbs which have the ability to enhance the immune system and protect against cancer. There are so many more but time does not permit us to go into this subject any further.

Studies have shown that exercise plays a major role in preventing certain types of cancer deaths especially colon cancer. Men and women who are physically fit have lower death rates from cancer. Michele Wolf reports in the October 1993 issue of "American Health", of a study of more than 10,000 men and 3000 women examined at the Institute of Aerobics Research in Dallas. This study showed that those who exercised regularly and were most fit on the treadmill test had a much lower rate of cancer deaths than those who were unfit. The study followed those individuals for a period of eight years and cancer deaths were very low amongst this group.[15] Evidence indicates that exercise does protect against colon cancer.

Dr. Wolf further reports that exercise for women, particularly during the teenage and young adult years, proves a lower rate of breast cancer and other

15 Ibid., 265.

hormone-related cancers of the reproductive organs.[16] Other studies done at Harvard School of Public Health under the direction of Dr. Rose Frisch found that among nearly 45,400 female college graduates, those who had been athletes or who worked out periodically had a much lower rate of developing cancer of the breast than did nonathletes. Those who were not athletically inclined nor who worked-out had higher rates of cancers of the uterus, ovary, cervix and vagina.[17]

Exercise reduces the risk of cancer in women and enables them to receive a lower dose of estrogen. Estrogen has been known to stimulate the growth of cells in the breasts and reproductive organs. It is known that physically active women can change the hormone ratio and reduce body fat. One third of estrogen before menopause is produced by body fat, consequently, it stands that leaner women will have less of this cancer stimulating hormone.[18]

Dr. Wolf adds that exercise may help fight other forms of cancer since it has the ability to boost the functioning of the immune system. It encourages two types of immune system cells: natural killer (NK) cells and macrophages which appear to inhibit tumor growth. If a tumor is growing, exercise will not stop the growth but may prevent the malignant cells from spreading. At this time we do not know how much exercise is needed to prevent the growth of cancer.

---

16 Ibid., 265.

17 Ibid., 265.

18 Ibid., 265.

Cancer rates differ appreciably in other parts of the world. This suggest to us that diet does play a significant role in cancer. Diets that contain foods with high levels of carbohydrates and cholesterol are not good for cancer prevention. Diets high in Vitamin E, C, Beta-carotene, fiber and other necessary nutrients aid in the prevention of cancer. Diets high in Vitamin C and fibre appear to help in the prevention of cancer and also help prevent heart disease. Adding Vitamin E to the diet, definitely helps in reducing not only the risk of cancer but heart disease.

Cancer specialist, Dr. Keith Block of Evanston, Illinois believes that diet is a critical factor in health and that what people eat makes a definite difference in the body's ability to resist disease. He also believes that diet will help us maintain good health. His diet for cancer patients consists of whole cereal grains, vegetables, legumes, fruits, nuts and seeds, soy foods, fish and free-range poultry. On his diet he restricts or even eliminates dairy products, eggs, red meats, refined sugar, caffeinated or alcoholic beverages, processed foods, no hydrogenated oils, and even some vegetables in the night shade family such as eggplant and green peppers.[19]

Dr. Block's diet is very similar to the diets recommended by the American Cancer Society, the National Cancer Institute, the American Academy of Sciences and the American Heart Association. Each of these groups believe that these diets have some

---

19 Ibid., 272.

preventive value in protecting against cancer and coronary heart disease.

As we have stressed earlier in this book that a positive mental attitude is necessary in enjoying life but now it is stressed in helping to overcome cancer. The mental state affects the outcome of cancer therapy and can assist the physician in making treatment more affective. Many now concede that a positive mental attitude can minimize the negative side effects of medical treatments such as chemotherapy and may even assist in it's cure.

We now know that we can change the body by learning how to deal with what we feel. Studies have shown that as we deal with pain and seek help, the body receives the message that living is more desirable than dying. According to Dr. Berni Siegel, this will actually encourage the immune system to respond positively. Dr. Siegel is a surgeon and a wholistic practitioner who has seen countless so called terminal patients turned around for the better. In his book, "Love, Medicine & Miracles", he relates actual cases of individuals being turned back from the edge to a full joyous life of experiencing radiant health.

When dealing with cancer, it is necessary to mobilize all of the person's forces such as the mental, emotional, physical and spiritual against the disease. Through regular group support meetings, nutritional counseling, exercise, prayer, visualization and a good trusting relationship with their physician, patients can then see themselves as getting well. The foundation has been laid and their patient than can turn from illness to anticipating a full recovery no matter what the odds might be.

We cannot under estimate the need of positive therapy while dealing with cancer and it's ramifications. Whether one uses prayer or meditation to help control pain, it must be done with the belief that each and every moment the individual is getting better and total recovery is possible.

At times cancer patients will experience negative emotions which is also an important component of the healing process. It is known that patients who repressed their emotions with their physicians, died substantially earlier than those who expressed themselves openly. The survivors consistently questioned their physicians and told them exactly how they felt. Those who have died early, according to the Psychologist Leonard Derogatis in a study of 35 women with metastatic breast cancer, found that these women had a poor relationship with their doctors. They often practiced denial and other psychological defenses.[20]

In other words, in all of the cancer literature we read that the expressing of both positive and negative emotions is a necessary part of the healing process. Of course, this does not go down with many physicians who come out of the old school of thought. Again it should be reiterated that patients who expressed themselves out lived those who did not.

---

20 Ibid., 273.

Although we have talked about vitamins in the previous chapters, it behooves us to discuss some new findings concerning Vitamin B6. Vitamin B6 is now considered to be one of the promising vitamins beneficial in the treatment of cancer. Dr. Hans Ladner and Dr. Richard Salkeld, German and Swiss researchers, have studied the effects of B6 on a clinical trial basis by treating cancer patients with this vitamin. The results were most impressive. This vitamin was given over a seven week period to 210 endometrial cancer patients, aged 45 to 65. Notice that these patients had a 15 percent improvement in the five-year survival rates as compared to the 105 patients who did not have the Vitamin B6 available to them. Again there were no side effects from B6 supplementation.[21] Vitamin B6 has proven effective in inhibiting melanoma cancer cells.

A research team cited in the book "Essential Nutrients in Carcinogenesis", developed a topical cream that showed a significant reduction of subcutaneous cancer nodules and regression of cutaneious papules. This may lead to several new forms of treatment for skin cancer.

Patients taking antioxidants while taking chemotherapy have lived longer than those who did not take vitamins and minerals. In particular this has been seen in reference to small cell cancer of the lungs. Patients taking vitamins, minerals and herbs have a

---

21 Ibid., 275.

much easier time while receiving radiation or chemotherapy.

We now know that both conventional and alternative therapies do extend patients' lives while being given at the same time. It also has been seen that cancer patients often do better when conventional therapies are necessary because their outlook makes them significantly more responsive to the disease itself. Physical and mental health of patients receiving wholistic healing while taking chemotherapy improved substantially. In other words, there is every indication that alternative therapies have much to offer and the medical profession needs to be more open to what is being offered.

# CHAPTER THIRTEEN

# A NEW THIN YOU

If we are attempting to lose weight we need to take a view of what wholistic healthy people eat. They eat all the essential foods they need in proper proportions so as not to gain weight. According to the Prevention Magazine, about 60 percent of Americans consume an excessive amount of unnecessary and wrong types of foods. It is now believed that 64 million Americans are overweight. This was determined through the use of insurance charts and company tables that dealt with age, sex and body build. The Louis Harris and Associates conducted this survey during 1993 for the Prevention Magazine. In my opinion, you can't go by insurance tables to find out what your correct weight ought to be. Nevertheless, it gives information about what we need and that is; that Americans are fatter now than at any other previous time in the history of this nation. It would appear that Americans are making less of an attempt to curb their wrong eating habits and continue to indulge in too much sugar and fast foods. In 1976, 125 pounds of sugar was consumed per person in the United States. In the year 1990, 140 pounds of sugar was consumed by each person. May we be delivered from this intake of poison! It also would appear that Americans are not taking their vitamins and minerals as they should since heart disease and cancer are on the increase. We need to adopt weight-loss programs consistent with the basics of alternative medicine, proper diet, sufficient exercise and a positive mental attitude. These are all things which have been covered in previous chapters but will be dealt with in this chapter on finding a New Thin You. Diets don't work! I've tried through the years to lose weight only to gain more back than which I actually lost. If you're thinking of trying a diet, don't! Get that idea out of your head. All of us must adopt a Christian wholistic approach to eating. You can rest assured that with this approach to a New Thin You, it will come about. Again, it is a lifestyle change. We should not be surprised that in such an affluent society as America, where food is so very abundant and where most people can easily buy food, that we have become a nation burdened by fat. This is a major health problem that must be dealt with or we are going to continue in obesity. Obesity must be considered a disease like any other since it eventually will kill the body. A disease is a disharmony and an imbalance in the body, and like all diseases, obesity is the result of poor choices in food selection. We just haven't been taught how to put together an eating program that will best suit our needs.

Let's take a brief look at some of the effects over-weight and obesity have upon the human body. For example, carrying 20, 30 or 40 pounds or even more all day around with you requires much additional energy and food intake. It's like carrying a couple of cement blocks on your back, hips or legs around with you all day long. It places a tremendous burden on the heart and joints of the body. The extra weight stimulates the person to eat more which causes a self-defeating, fat-sustaining life style. It is one that can be changed with God's help.

Here are some of the changes in the body connected with obesity. Adipose tissue, consisting of large round cells which store fat and cholesterol, increases in quantity, supported by collagen tissue, and fed by additional blood vessels.[1] Blood lipids are increased, especially triglycerides. The sugar in alcoholic beverages causes an additional increase in the production of triglycerides. At the same time the bad cholesterol, LDL will in turn be increased, thus the good cholesterol, HDL will diminish. The person is set up for heart disease. Remember, each pound of fat on the body requires more blood vessels. This puts additional strain on the heart.

I do realize that facts like these certainly are not inspiring but the truth must be known. You are on a journey while you're reading this book and this book can bring great health benefits if you will take the

---

1 Dr. Bernard Jensen, <u>Slender Me Naturally</u>, (Bernard Jensen, Ph.D., Escondido, CA. 1986), 4.

time to put into practice the suggestions found here. You may have a goal to lose weight and become a thinner you. If that is the case, this chapter will greatly bless you.

The cardiovascular system, especially the heart, suffers from overwork. Excess weight increases the chance of heart disease and high blood pressure. In addition to this, it greatly enhances the increase of atherosclerosis, the fatty deposits in the linings of arterial walls that will reduce the artery diameter. It does restrict the blood flow and can lead to a heart attack or stroke.

The lymphatic system also suffers from too many extra pounds. The lymphatic system is a vast network of vessels throughout the body that contains about 45 pints of fluid. Unlike the circulatory system, the lymphatic system has no "heart" to pump it through its system of vessels. As the muscles contract, the lymph is squeezed along the muscles during the course of normal activity. As individuals gain weight, there is less movement of the lymph. Since the lymph carries nutrients to the cells and waste products from them, the result is less effective removal of waste and toxins from this system. The end result is an environment that is set up for disease.[2]

As a person gains excess weight more oxygen is needed. At the same time the lungs have a fixed level of capacity. Since the lungs can't meet the new demands being placed upon them the body goes into

---

2  Ibid., 5.

an oxygen deficit. The cells and tissues will all suffer because of the new demands being placed upon the lungs. As abdominal fat presses against the lungs and limits breathing, there is a further reduction of the required oxygen need for the body.

As a result of this every organ of the body suffers with a lower level of functioning. Glands and tissues requiring sufficient oxygen are adversely effected. If there is a respiratory disease in the body, such as asthma, complications can be most serious.

When a person is obese, the fatty tissue throughout the body tends to make the bowel flaccid, leading to prolapse of the transverse colon, balloon-like conditions and bowel pockets. Also, there is underactivity of the bowel and the ever ensuing problem of constipation. Often the stomach cavity is displaced and pushes into the chest. More toxic waste builds up in the bowel only to be eventually absorbed into the blood stream. Overweight also effects every organ of the digestive system causing it to become inherently weak.

Overweight people suffer unduly with greater wear and tear on their joints, especially in cases of arthritis.[3] Spinal problems such as slipped or ruptured disks are more common amongst obese people. These painful conditions further reduce the physical activity of the overweight individuals. The end product is that these individuals tend to gain more weight, thus compounding the problems.

---

3  Ibid., 5.

The liver and gallbladder are greatly overworked because of the lowered physical activity, bowel underactivity and lymphatic congestion. The liver is especially affected since it is not able to perform its many tasks. One study showed that 88 percent of 215 people operated on for gallbladder disease and stones were overweight.[4]

Television and overweight seem to go hand in hand. People sit before the television many hours a day, seeing beautiful young slender bodies of both sexes advertising all kinds of products. This unconsciously causes guilt on the part of the overweight viewer who than desires unwittingly to even eat more.

At the same time television programs are offering countless food products for sale at the local grocery store that usually are high in fat and sodium. Viewers are enticed to buy these products but are not told about the amount of fat and cholesterol contained in them.

If you go to the grocery store you will find by the check out counters the latest tabloids advertising the newest fad diet which promises instant success with a tremendous weight loss. Literally every year millions of Americans go through starvation diets trying to shed those unwanted pounds only to gain them back. The only problem is they usually gain back more than they lose. They may even take special diet pills, protein powers, eat only fruits and try to stay away from fattening foods. After a few weeks of this arduous

---

4   Ibid., 6.

attempt they fall back into their same old eating habits. We call this the yo-yo approach to slimming. It just doesn't work and there is a better way to reduce.

It is estimated that at any given time approximately 40 million Americans are on diets. Many have tried the latest fad diets with some success only to regain the weight they lost. It is known that on some of the fad diets people have died because of ingesting too much protein, raising their blood cholesterol level to an extraordinary high level thus bringing on a sudden heart attack.

Some of the new powder diets provide only 330 to 500 calories a day which becomes a starvation or fasting diet. According to Dr. Bernard Jensen, these diets produce muscle waste, water loss, nutritional imbalance, endocrine system imbalance, fatigue and other most serious health problems which can occur from these unnatural diets.[5]

The average individual is simply not informed about food, nutrition and the functioning of the body to safely carry out a low fat or an extremely low calorie diet program. It is known that very heavy people who lose weight too rapidly often die shortly after their tremendous weight loss.

If fad diets, protein powders and diet pills were the answer to overweight, it would have been resolved a long time ago. It is the person that must make an intelligent decision to change his lifestyle of eating.

---

5  Ibid., 9.

A tendency to gain weight easily may be due to numerous inherited conditions. There are many glands, nerves and organs involved in the process of digestion and if there is an inherent weakness in any one of them, the fatty tissue production could be a potential problem. Inherent weakness can be overcome by proper eating, exercise and a wholesome mental attitude.

The glands and organs that have to do with fat metabolism are the hypothalamus, pituitary gland, thyroid gland, pancreas, adrenals, sex glands, liver, gallbladder and small intestine. Should there be an inherent weakness in any one of these organs, we could have a definite problem with weight control.

Each person metabolizes his or her foods differently. Some metabolize their food faster than others. Some have an abundance of digestive enzymes while others do not. Some have very good mental attitudes while others do not. All of these factors must be taken into consideration when evaluating weight gain or loss.

One of the main problems with a fad diet is that it throws some of the glands off balance. When weight is lost too fast the thyroid gland slows down to accommodate this loss and the resultant effect is slower metabolism. At the same time, the hypothalamus turns on the hunger "switch" causing even a greater craving for food. The brain stays tuned until all the weight that has been lost is regained and even more added to it. These diets are absolutely useless since the brain works the way that it does.

The pituitary is the master gland of the body and of the endocrine glandular system. When the pituitary is disturbed by a growth on or near it, this can be a contributing cause of weight gain. The pituitary is connected to the hypothalamus of the brain. The appetite center is located in the hypothalamus.[6] Please understand that the appetite center is associated with the blood levels of various nutrients.

All of these things are very important since an imbalance of the sex hormone estrogen, can spur obesity, and the adrenal hormone aldosterone, controls water retention in the body.[7] The amount of salt that is used in foods affects the aldosterone level in the body. Very low calorie diets dramatically alter the nutrient levels and balances in the body. This will disrupt the glandular system, leading to abnormal weight gain. According to Dr. Bernard Jensen, the short-term success in weight loss leads to long-term failure.[8]

Weight gain is often associated with menopause. It is a most frustrating experience for a woman to go through. The body chemistry is so very complex it becomes difficult to know how to treat the problem of menopausal weight gain in women.

Menopausal weight gain is often associated with adjustments in the endocrine system. Such herbs as black cohosh and licorice are beneficial during

---

6   Ibid., 16.

7   Ibid., 16.

8   Ibid., 17.

menopause, and men will find that ginseng and fo ti tieng will help balance the male glands.[9]

What you think or don't thing can actually affect weight gain or weight loss. Many people eat out of habit, having the notion that they must eat three square meals a day. These people may not even need that amount of food to sustain themselves but, because of poor nutritional upbringing, they consume this every day of their lives.

There are times when we have food cravings which will present a challenge not to give in to them. It is best to get outside and do some walking. We must do anything we can to get our minds off of the food. My wife sips on an apple cider vinegar, honey and warm water drink to alleviate the craving of some sweet that is in the kitchen cupboard. Food can be addictive!! Many people find that food is pulling at them all the time like a bull with a ring in its nose. They have to have it or they go crazy.

Some people lust after their food. They literally breath it in as fast as they can. If you want to see what I am talking about just go to an all you can eat restaurant. People return to the buffet table for a second and third helping and eat everything on their plate. This would be expected of farmers who work all day putting fence posts in place. People just don't have the discipline to say "no" to their desires for food.

---

9   Ibid., 17.

Some people overeat because they are bored or depressed. Some eat since they feel they are not loved. In this case food takes the place of a lover. A survey was done over television some years ago and it showed that 87 percent of teenage girls did not like their bodies. Just what does a thought like this do to the appetite center? When we study the extreme effects of emotion and thought in anorexia and bulimia cases it is evident that what people think has much to do with how they eat. What people think also will determine the amount of food that is eaten. One of the ways of losing unwanted pounds is to start thinking positively about yourself and your circumstances.

Research through the years has shown that the brain "decides" on how much fat our bodies actually need and we eat until we have attained that weight. To me this is pure "nonsense". If this was true many people in the third world would be over-weight like the Americans, but they are not because they lack food. Many in the third world actually starve on a daily basis. We are fat because we eat the wrong things and too much of them.

It is my opinion that the body gets accustomed to the amount of weight that it is carrying whether it is the correct amount of weight or not. Remember that fat is not dead matter. It has blood vessels and nerves running through it. It is estimated that for each pound of fat there are 600 feet of additional blood vessels. Fat affects the blood chemistry and the amount of work the heart has to do.

If the brain considers a certain amount of fat natural to the body, it goes into shock if there is a rapid weight loss. Somehow the brain considers this an imbalance of body chemistry. As this occurs, the metabolism drops to conserve energy and to keep functions going at a coma reduced level. This accounts for the plateau that many dieters come to, not understanding why they can't lose more. The brain stores up a long-term hunger which is geared for additional weight gain after the diet has ended. Any permanent weight loss program must take this into account in order to be successful and not gain back extra weight.[10]

Remember that overweight problems boil down to eating too much of the wrong foods. When we eat the right foods we will see a natural weight loss occur. If we eat the wrong foods, especially fatty foods, we definitely will gain unwanted pounds. If we do not consume the correct foods, we will develop chemical imbalances. Since we have already considered the digestive process in this book, we will not go into this again.

We cannot over estimate the need of taking care of the bowel. Bowel regularity and colon hygiene are very important in preventing disease and maintaining a healthy body. A sluggish bowel, constipation and bowel irregularity have two consequences that encourage obesity.[11] The longer waste remains in the bowel, the more fat and cholesterol are absorbed into the blood stream. Again, this is also true of toxic poisons that the

---

10 Ibid., 20.

11 Ibid., 22.

body is attempting to rid itself of. If the toxic poisons should get past the liver (our great detoxifier of the body), they will be placed in the weakest organs of the body. Toxic settlements have a tendency to lower the metabolism of tissues where they have settled, and nearly every time weight gain will appear in those areas. Once again, if we desire to loss weight we must take good care of the colon.

It takes 3,500 calories of food to build a pound of fat and it will take 3,500 calories of energy to burn up that same pound.[12] The best way to lose weight is to burn up more calories per day than you actually eat. This means that we will need to exercise more if the weight is to come off from our frame. Eating less is the best way to accomplish your desired weight goal. Eating less but eating quality food with less fat will bring definite positive results.

It takes more calories to maintain an overweight body than one that is at its ideal weight. One can expect an energy lag as the diet is changed to more wholesome foods. The less junk food like coffee, alcohol and other valueless food you take in, the more abundant energy will be available but you will experience a temporary energy lag.

The brain doesn't know that you're changing your diet, but sees the lower food intake as starvation which triggers an inherent survival mechanism into action. The thyroid slows down the use of energy throughout the entire body. Metabolism slows down to balance

---

12 Ibid., 29.

with the decreased food consumption. This is the initiating factor which brings on an energy lag. As this is going on, the brain stores in its memory the fact that the body is losing weight which must be regained later.[13]

Another most important element in the diet are the enzymes in the body which have been busy building and maintaining the fat cells that are still there. These enzymes are no longer "employed" as such. These "unemployed" enzymes are an important part in both the relentless hunger response end of the diet and the consequent weight-gain effect.[14]

Our bodies are fat because we eat to much fat. There is a proper way to take in fats. We are able to obtain all the fats we need when we use foods such as whole milk, eggs, avocados, nuts, nut butters and other natural foods.[15]

Our ultimate goal is to lose weight. If you think that you can do it on a diet, you probably will lose weight. At the same time, the odds are against you and you will gain the weight back. Stay away from diets and choose a healthy lifestyle of eating and see your weight drop off slowly but permanently. Your new eating habits will consist of selecting foods that are natural, whole, fresh and alive. You will not want to eat those dead foods that have no living enzymes in them. Stay away from all products that contain white sugar and white flour.

---

13 Ibid., 29.

14 Ibid., 29.

15 Ibid., 30.

The rule of thumb is that all packaged foods and all foods containing chemical additives should be avoided. The processing of these foods have destroyed them of valuable nutrients and since any added chemicals are a potential danger to health, we should not eat this kind of lifeless foods. Stay with natural foods, whole, pure and as close to being raw as possible. Be very cautious about frozen foods because these too have had chemicals added to them.

As you change your diet to one of being more natural or totally vegetarian, weight will begin to come off with-out the effort of dieting. Avoid fried foods and those fried in hydrogenated oils. The body has a difficult time getting rid of hydrogenated fats.

Get the junk foods out of your house and you won't be tempted to eat them. After a while your taste will change and you will desire a natural diet. You will feel better and you will certainly look better.

Learn to eat lots of raw vegetables. You will lose excess weight on such a food program. Use fresh fruits as your snacks between meals. Eat carrots, celery, radishes, sliced cucumbers, tomatoes and other raw vegetables on your new eating regimen. Try to eat five to six vegetables a day and you will become radiant with new energy and vigor. Stop eating white bread, white sugar and whole milk since these only add to additional weight and ill health.

You can succeed on this new lifestyle change. Weight will decrease gradually and your waist line will definitely become smaller. Give it a good try! You have nothing to lose but weight!

# CHAPTER FOURTEEN

# THE JOY OF JUICING

Juicing should occupy a good part of any health building regime. Juices are easily digested and most pleasant to drink. They give new vitality and are full of live enzymes so necessary for good health. There are countless combinations that can be created specially for numerous ailments. There are combinations for heating up the body and cooling down the body. Juicing is one of the most wonderful health programs known to mankind.

We need to have an understanding of various raw juices, tonics, and teas and what they will or will not do for the human body. If your body is catarrh-laden, raw fruit juices will stir up toxins and acids but do very little to eliminate the waste from the body. Vegetable juices are excellent for elimination of toxins while fruit juices are very good for their vitamin content. The advantage to juicing is that the juice will contain the concentrated form of vitamins and minerals. Please keep in mind that we must have fibre in our diet and we get this from whole fruits and vegetables.

Fresh juices should be taken between meals, but if you are juice fasting, they may be taken at regular meal times. Remember to sip your juice and never gulp it down. Enjoy the taste and the fragrance of what you're drinking.

Juices that elevate the body temperature and maintain body heat are known as thermades, while drinks that reduce body heat and temperature are known as frescades.[1] All fruit juices that contain cooling acids such as formic citric and acetic acid are especially good for warm or hot weather. If you're in the tropics, the local fruits can be juiced and used to cool down the body. Adding certain herbs, plants and leaves will contribute to the cooling effect. Remember, if too much perspiration occurs on hot days, this can become a contributing factor to summer illness. Formic acid in the body can be obtained from juicing.

Vegetable juices are high in potassium and may be helpful as a laxative. At the same time, if these are used over a long period of time, they can cause digestive problems. Drinking too much blackberry juice can be constipating since it is very high in iron. Fruit juices are true vitalizers since they contain a high level of vitamins. One of the most wonderful aspects of juicing is that fresh juices have an antiseptic property to assist in the battle against bacteria and viruses.

---

1  Dr. Bernard Jensen, Ph.D., <u>Food Healing For Man</u>, (Bernard Jensen Enterprises, Escondido, California, 1983), 298.

Blackberries, found in Oregon, Washington, Northern California, Virginia, Michigan and Tennessee contain a substantial amount of iron more so than the domestic type berries. Both forms of these are constipating.[2]

Wild cherries contain the same acids as blackberries. Phosphoric, tannic, and tartaric acids are abundant in these berries. Domestic cherries contain a certain gum which benefits the bowels. Both domestic and wild cherries contain numerous salts needed by the tissues, especially potassium. They function as a laxative to a stomach low in acid.[3]

Prunes and prune juice act as a laxative to many people. Prunes are full of potassium, phosphorus, calcium and sodium.

Strawberries are a mild laxative. They contain malic acid, sodium, potassium, calcium, phosphorus, sulphur, iron and a small amount of evonymin.[4]

Black and blue huckleberries have similar qualities as blueberries. Their juice is most refreshing and very good for you.

Blueberry juice is full of phosphoric, tartaric, and tannic acids. They are also high in potassium, calcium and magnesium. It makes a wonderful drink if it is diluted with spring water or distilled water.

---

2  Ibid., 298.

3  Ibid., 298.

4  Ibid., 299.

Pineapple juice is recommended for throat infection and other throat ailments. It contains sodium, calcium, magnesium and iodine.

Mangoes contain gallic acid. This acid functions as a mild disinfectant and binds to the bowel walls. The juice of a mango counteract perspiration, reduces excess body heat and acts to eliminate unpleasant odors from the body. The main elements found in the mangoe are potassium, calcium and chlorine.

Apple juice makes a most excellent beverage. It contains potassium, sodium, magnesium, phosphorus and several fruit acids, especially malic acid.[5] Apple juice may be mixed with other juices whether they are sweet or bitter. Apple juice is good for an acid stomach since it contains pectin.

Watermelon juice is a good kidney cleanser. The white rind of the melon is rich in sodium, and very good for the stomach and bowel. The green skin which is usually thrown away, is rich in chlorophyll. Chlorophyll acts as a blood cleanser and detoxifier. Watermelon seeds act as a mild diuretic for the kidneys while the pink meat contains silicon, calcium, and sufficient fruit sugar to supply energy for the whole body. Do not eat watermelon or drink its juice at least within one half hour of eating other foods. Melon should not be consumed with other foods. The rich benefit of these melons are greatly reduced if combined with other foods. A point to remember about eating any melon is: eat it alone or leave it alone!

---

5   Ibid., 299.

Grape juice is high in magnesium and phosphorus, and if the grape skin is juiced at the same time, it will be high in potassium. Grapes are also high in iron. This juice is very good as a blood purifier and acts as a laxative.

Now let's take some time and look at the vegetable kingdom. Vegetables function as builders and toners and are wonderful sources of chemical elements. The roles of fruits and vegetables at times run concurrent, meaning they function in a similar manner.

Iceberg or head lettuce has so very little nutritional value. It is virtually worthless. Leaf lettuces are much better for you since they are full of chlorophyll and various vitamins and some minerals.

Onions are very good for all of us. The juice of an onion stimulates the kidneys, lungs and throat. Onions are full of an oil called allyl sulphide. At the same time, the minerals found in the onion are most beneficial for the body. Those minerals are potassium, calcium, phosphorus, iron, sulphur and silicon.[6] Garlic and leeks are members of the same family and have similar properties. Garlic functions as a natural antiseptic and antibiotic, which is an excellent aid during the cold and flu seasons. The sulphur in garlic and leeks works as a stirring element and is known to penetrate the cells in a most profound way.

Celery and parsley contain a very small amount of apiol. Apiol is known to work on the sexual system.

---

6  Ibid., 301.

When celery and parsley are taken in juice form, the nervous system is toned and sexual function is greatly improved. Apiol has also been known to assist during menstruation to relieve some of the unpleasant symptoms. Since celery juice is high in sodium, it has been known to relieve the symptoms of rheumatism and arthritis. Celery is also high in sodium and it brings back the chemical balance to the joints.

Carrot juice is delicious to drink and is very high in pro-vitamin A, this is the carotene that is transformed into Vitamin A in the body. The juice of carrots is full of potassium, silicon and chlorine salts.[7] A combination of carrot juice and spinach, will supply the body with most of the needed body salts. Carrot juice is most beneficial for the treatment of chronic disease. It supplies the body with live enzymes and beta carotene which helps the body restore itself.

Spinach juice is considered the queen of all the greens. It is full of potassium, sodium, calcium, magnesium, phosphorus, sulphur and silicon. There is a very small amount of iron but the plant is most helpful in creating health. I have seen it do wonders for the chronically ill.

Tomato juice is a good source of potassium, phosphorus, calcium and numerous fruit essences. A tomato is a fruit and not a vegetable. It is excellent for the blood and is known to cool the body.

---

7  Ibid., 301.

One of my favorite juices is that of the cucumber. It acts as a mild tonic, a refreshing drink during the summer and a strong sedative at night.[8] There are bitter oils in the rind of a cucumber so peel it before juicing. Cut off a small piece near one end and rub the two cut surfaces together in a circular motion. The foam that builds up is eliminating the bitter oils from the inner lining and leaves a sweeter taste. I used to watch my mother foam up the cucumbers and never knew why. Then peel the cucumber and juice it.

The dandelion, a flower that most people dislike, is full of trace minerals. It is most beneficial for building up the body since it is full of iron and other necessary trace minerals. Dandelion can be an excellent tonic and function as a laxative.

Beet juice must be diluted with water since it is very strong. It contains a small amount of ergot and betin, and works wonderfully as a liver cleanser. It is full of potassium, sodium, phosphorus, magnesium, and a touch of iron.

Coffee and tea are high in caffeine which has a most negative effect on the body. Ordinary black tea contains gallic, tannic, phosphoric, carbonic and boheic acids. Quinic is found in coffee. Regular coffee drinking has been linked to a higher rate of heart disease, and it encourages too much acid in the stomach.

Cabbage is very high in many organic salts and in brassidic acid, which is excellent for asthma victims.

---

8  Ibid., 301.

The cabbage family includes cauliflower, kale, sea kale, broccoli, savoy, sprouts, kohlrabi, shallot and red cabbage. All of these are rich in organic salts and full of potassium. In Poland, where cabbage is eaten raw or cooked, the incidences of colon cancer are very small as compared to the West.

Cabbage juice can be combined with those of other vegetables to create an excellent drink for numerous health ailments. There is only one little problem with cabbage and other members of the cabbage family, they create a lot of gas. This should not stop one from drinking these most healing drinks.

In our previous descriptions of the constituents of fruits and vegetable juices, we have attempted to show you the profound value juicing can have on the promotion of personal health. If you truly wish to become younger, start juicing as soon as possible. Not only can fresh fruits and vegetables provide vitamins and minerals, they can also assist one in losing weight. Much of the vitamins and minerals found in raw vegetables are held within the fiber. The fiber is that part of the vegetable that the body cannot use and which the body naturally expunges. However, when a fruit or vegetable is properly juiced, these normally inaccessible vitamins and minerals are released and easily absorbed into the blood stream.

There must be a word of caution when juicing berries. The natural sugars in barriers are held within the fibre. When eaten raw, many calories are not absorbed but when juiced, the sugars and excess calories are easily absorbed into the blood stream. So watch how much you are drinking because you could be putting on needless pounds, which only later have to be exercised off.

Always, when making your own juice, make sure to remove seeds and stems from your fruits and vegetables. Remember apple seeds and carrot roots contain toxins that have been shown to be harmful to the human body.

It's alright to juice lemon and lime skins with your fruit, but others such as oranges, grapefruits and kiwi skins definitely need to be removed before juicing.

The white part of oranges and grapefruits just below the peel is known as a bioflavonoid and is very rich in vitamins. Make sure that this white part is juiced and not thrown into the trash.

Here is a little tip for you. It's best to drink your fresh fruit juice through a straw because sipping drinks through a straw gives more pleasure to your taste buds.

Now let's take a brief look at herbal teas. Herbal teas, including the wide variety of teas that do not contain caffeine or sugar, are excellent for those desiring to lose weight. If they are hot or cold, they are perfect for quenching the thirst. When herbal tea is consumed cold, it functions just like water and fat is flushed out of the body. Diet herbal teas have been used in China for hundreds of years since some actually reduce sugar and fat absorption while the digestive process speeds up.

If you desire to flush out fat from your body, make sure that herbal teas are a part of your regime. Use your favorite tea since it will prevent boredom and help you lose further calories.

Here are a few teas which are most healing for the body. Peppermint tea contains pimenthol which is beneficial for the nerves. It is good for fermentation and for gas which has been generated from starches and sugars.

Catnip tea is rich in potassium. It works as a gas driver and expulsion agent. This tea is especially good for those who have problems with constipation. If the diet has been high in milk and dairy products, this tea will cause a normal flow of the bowels.

Sage tea contains salviol and tennin which function as binding agents in the bowels. It helps relieve diarrhea, and is known as a very good tonic. Adding a little lemon juice makes it more palpable to the taste buds.

Thyme tea is a bacteriocidal, tonic, calming and helps to relieve itching. Thyme juice may be added to other juices with great results.[9]

Wintergreen tea is binding but still acts as a tonic. It is excellent in counteracting uric acid and gout. By the way, my grandfather drank this tea every winter when it was so terribly cold in Michigan. As a little boy, he introduced me to this wonderful tea. My grandfather

---

9   Ibid., 302.

lived to be an elderly gentleman always telling me about his winter medicines, herbs and teas.

The water of cloves contains caryophyllin and eugenin, and is very good for infection and toothache. It acts as a tonic and rids the body of various types of bacteria.

Sarsaparilla drinks are very good for kidney and bowel stimulation. There are several types of saponins, a volatile oil and a resin have been found in sarsaparilla.

Ginger is aromatic and excellent for driving gas out of the body. Ginger has been used by the American Indians for hundreds of years as a healer of various digestive problems.

Sassafras is made from bark. It is known to be full of tannin and also an aromatic oil. It makes a delightful tea which helps eliminate catarrh, purifies the blood and assists in digestion. It is known to ward of insects.[10]

Juniper berries are very abundant in the Southwest of the United States and for years they have been used as a mild diuretic and to tone up the reproductive system. Supposedly it enhances one's sexual life. They have additional properties to cleanse the liver and the blood. There must be a word of caution here about using them as a tea, as they can be very hard on the kidneys. Use this tea for only a few days at a time since it could do harm.

---

10 Ibid., 302.

In this chapter we have had a limited description on fruits and vegetables in relationship to juicing. We have had some information about herbal teas which should encourage you to want to change your way of eating. If these things are taken seriously, it can only be a great blessing to you and your family. Give it a chance in your life. You will feel better and even begin to look younger.

## CHAPTER FIFTEEN

# STAYING YOUNGER LONGER BY KNOWING YOUR ANTIOXIDANTS

We now have the knowledge of specific nutrients that will enable the average person to remain youthful for a longer period of time. Taking necessary antioxidants and fasting will strengthen the immune system. Specific nutrients are able to activate sluggish glands, enhance the immune system and aid in repairing biological assaults against the body itself.

In chapter seven, we discussed briefly the theory of free radicals which is the real cause of aging. There is more than enough research to substantiate the damage that free radicals can have on the body. These are the primary cause of aging. They are produced in the body during metabolism. Their life span is very short but can be most destructive. They specialize in destroying cell membranes. Free radicals are molecules which have an unstable charge. They are most active in the presence of other molecules.

Most books on nutrition state unequivocally that it is during the oxidizing process that the free radicals attack lipids (fats) to form compounds called aldehydes and other negative oxidative by-products. These in turn will react with proteins and generate cross-linked aggregates. These then will flow through the blood system and eventually wind up entering the cell membranes to cause injury. Within the cell are mitochondria which appear like little cushions. Inside the mitochondria are two small membranes called cristae which are the targets for the free radicals. As the cristae are assaulted, they promote premature aging.[1]

Once this reaction begins in any place of the body, the end product can be devastating. The body's organs, cells and systems begin to deteriorate. It is a slow process that can even begin in the late teen years if the diet is poor. The process can be measured and felt on a gradual basis.

There are a group of nutrients known as antioxidants that can bolster your immune response which will add in resisting the onslaught of the free radicals. These nutrients work like scavengers in the body, and as they sweep through the system they collect the corrosive fragments and roots and push them out of the system. Please note that these nutritional antioxidants slow up the accumulation of lipofuscin, the end product of free radical damage.[2]

---

1  Carlson Wade, <u>Nutritional Healers</u>, (Parker Publishing Company, West Nyake, N.Y., 1987), 241.

2  Ibid., 242.

When oxygen combines with such substances as fats, they eventually will become rancid. As this takes place, free radicals are formed. Antioxidants function to control and prevent this kind of rancidity. Antioxidants are really nutritional preservatives. They help regulate the oxidative risk which maintains an internal purity within the body. Consequently, your cells will stay younger longer.

All of us want to maintain health and youthfulness by protecting our cell membranes from the process of oxidation. Oxidation is devastating to the human body since it pits and corrodes the cell membranes. It is like rust corroding an old car bumper. It is a very serious process that leads to numerous degenerative diseases such as arthritis, cancer and some infections which are the result of free radical damage. The free radicals will attack your lymphocytes (white blood cells) that assist the immune system in fighting off viruses and other infectious agents.

Antioxidants work in helping to prevent free radical destruction of cell membranes. They are most therapeutic, protecting the cells against undesirable reactions with oxygen but allowing the good oxygen reactions to proceed without interruption.

Antioxidants form a group of cell protectors that put a damper on the destructive free radicals. They include Vitamin A, a nutrient which helps to suppress the malignancy of cultured cells transformed by the use of radiation, chemicals or viruses.[3]

---

3   Ibid., 244.

Vitamin A strengthens the epithelial cells. Epithelial cells line certain body cavities such as the mouth, throat, stomach, intestines, skin and the retina of the eyes.

Beta-carotene, another most excellent antioxidant, is partially converted into Vitamin A. Beta-carotene functions to strengthen the entire body system. Beta-carotene is found in vegetables that are red, yellow and dark green such as carrots, deep yellow squash, dark salad greens, sweet potato and broccoli. The fruit sources are apricot, cantaloupe, peach, nectarine and mango. Beta-carotene helps the body by protecting it from cellular toxicity and is a form of natural therapy against allergies.

The importance of Vitamin C as an antioxidant cannot be over emphasized. Vitamin C functions within the cell in a watery fluid. It soaks up free radicals forming two life saving compounds, dehydroascrobic acid and diketogulonic acid. It is believed that diketogulonic acid is a strong cancer fighting agent.[4] All of us know that when the common cold troubles us, Vitamin C helps boost up the immune system. It actually helps the lymphocytes to fight infection. There is some evidence that Vitamin C may help prevent the growth of human leukemia.

We cannot leave out Vitamin E which is one of the most important antioxidants that we have. It works as a scavenger, absorbing the dangerous oxidative by-products and flushing them out of the system. It is also involved in regulating health and aging. Vitamin

---

4  Ibid., 244.

E also boosts the immune system. It protects against the excessive production of lipofuscin, the biological age marker.[5]

The trace mineral, selenium, is considered to be a very powerful immune system stimulator. It triggers antibody production. Selenium controls the accumulation of lipofuscin, the aging pigment which interferes with cellular existence and rejuvenation. Selenium helps break down fats that can contribute to arteriosclerosis. Selenium is one little trace mineral you can't afford to exclude from your diet.

We are hearing so very much today about zinc, another necessary and most important trace mineral and a potent antioxidant, which boosts the immune function. Zinc is also necessary in that it helps the body in making protein. Zinc is important for every cell of the body because it assists the cells in reproduction.

It is so very important as Christians that we take good care of our bodies. Our bodies are the temple of the Holy Spirit. These temples need to be cared for with the best nutrition we can possible obtain.

We need to boost our resistance to the destructive free radicals with the proper foods that will supply all the antioxidants necessary for good health. If you're not able to find the foods that will provide all of the antioxidants on a daily basis, then do the next best thing. Go to a good health food store and buy supplements which will assist you on your diet regime.

---

5   Ibid., 245.

We must take a good look at the thymus gland since it may hold the key to rejuvenation. The thymus gland is a flat, pinkish-gray, two-lobed gland that lies behind the sternum and lungs in your chest. The thymus distributes and nourishes white blood cells. These cells are called lymphocytes which act as your body's defense against disease.

The thymus gland acts as a headquarters for what we call the killer T-cells or lymphocytes. When these cells meet a virus or other intruders in the body, they act as an antagonist and kill the invading enemy. It is known that cancer cells are destroyed by the killer T-cells. The T-cells actually gobble up harmful cells and wash them out of your body. If this gland should become weak, one of the main defense mechanisms in the body is critically affected and resistance to disease is greatly diminished.

The thymus gland is at its maximum size during our adolescent years. As we gradually grow older, the gland begins to shrink in size and the ability of the T-cells declines. Consequently, more disease appears as we become older.

It has been thought that the reduction of the size and function of the thymus gland was a major contributing factor in disease. At this present time we have the knowledge of nutrition to keep this gland at its peak performance even though it maybe smaller in size. Proper nutrition needed for this gland will help reduce the aging process. Once again, we come back to our old friend zinc, that trace mineral which cannot be over emphasized.

The thymus releases a hormone called thymosin. Thymosin helps to build immunity and resistance against aging. The thymus is a storehouse for zinc. If at any time the body is low in zinc, the function of the thymus is weakened. It is zinc that stimulates the thymus to release thymosin which in turn calls to action T-lymphocytes to do battle against age causing elements.

You can extend your life through proper nutrition. Not only will your life be extended, but the very quality of it will be greatly improved. Gerontology, which is the science of aging and old age itself, has proven that aging is definitely related to nutrition. With the use of the right nutrition and supplementation, many aspects of aging can be halted. At least many of the consequences of the process of aging can be prevented or slowed down substantially. It is believed that in the future, with the correct nutrition and vitamin-mineral therapy, aging may be abolished.

Today there is a great deal of talk about an over the counter product called DHEA. DHEA is short for dehydroepiandrosterone (D-hi-dro-ep-E-an-dro-stehr-own), a hormone made by the adrenal glands located just above the kidneys. There have been countless claims made about this product.

DHEA is not a new hormone that we have discovered. It was first found in 1934 and there have been countless articles written about it. There has been a great deal of interest about this hormone especially by wholistic practitioners.

DHEA is taking everything we've always assumed about getting older into a topsy-turvy position. We know that things we thought true thirty years ago may be in actual fact not true after all.

For years we were told just to accept the fact that our bodies and minds will run down and fall apart all over. Our scientists are telling us now we can actually live to be 120 years old and perhaps even longer.

Not only will we live longer but we add life to our years. The quality of life will improve if we take into consideration the need of vitamins, minerals and certain hormones to help slow the aging process.

DHEA can change the way we perceive old age. Being 70 or 80 or even 90 doesn't mean you have to be feeble or infirm. You can expect to laugh, love, feel good and look great even at an advanced age. The biblical age of 120 is now possible.

DHEA restores energy, improves your mood, increases your sex drive, reduced body fat and causes your skin to have a glow about it. We know that DHEA has a most positive effect on the immune system. There is evidence that DHEA helps those with chronic fatigue syndrome.

Scientists have known about DHEA for many years but have thought very little about it. In 1984, Dr. Norman Orentreich proved that DHEA production drops dramatically as we advance in age. Dr. Orentreich believes that this is the aging factor in promoting old age. In so many words, the less we have of it the quicker we age.[6]

This raised the question that, if we take more of it, will we slow down the aging process? Also, it is believed that by taking this hormone we can actually reverse the aging process.

The production of DHEA is at its peak during adolescence. When we reach about 20, the levels stay more or less constant until we reach the age of 45.

During your adulthood, it is believed that DHEA helps to regulate our moods, energy, strength, sex drive and even intelligence. Once an individual reaches his or her mid-40's to early 50's, DHEA production slows down and the wrinkles, sags, arches, and other signs of aging begin to take hold.

Studies have been done during the past ten years which indicate that, DHEA may in fact restore lost youthfulness. These studies were done on animals so not many people paid much attention to them. Scientists were most reluctant to recommend it for human beings. The reason was that they saw so much improvement in mice and other animals that they didn't want to give a false impression to the populace. At the same time, there was overwhelming evidence which could not be ignored.

In 1980, Dr. Arthur Schwartz of Temple University shocked a group of noted scientists by relating to them

6 Jim O'Brien, <u>Why Everyone's Talking about DHEA</u>, (Globe Communications Corp., Boca Raton, FL., 1997), 12.

the fascinating properties of DHEA. In his study, he added DHEA to the food of obese rats and found that it literally melted away their fat.[7] No one could understand how this could be but it was worth further investigation.

Dr. Schwartz related information about studies that were being done in Great Britain. Cancer specialists in England found that women with low levels of DHEA had higher rates of breast cancer than women with normal levels of the hormone. This link clearly suggested a connection between hormone levels and cancerous tumors of the breast.[8] At the same time much investigation would be needed to establish further evidence of the same.

Dr. Schwartz gave his rats injections of a powerful carcinogen that would normally cause tumor growth in a short period of time. Before doing this, he gave an injection of DHEA to each rat. Each rat that had been injected with DHEA remained cancer free.

There is a need for further study so that facts may be established beyond any shadow of doubt. Human studies must be done to substantiate the effects of DHEA on cancerous tumors.

In 1994, Dr. Samuel Yen of the University of California published an indepth study on the effectiveness of DHEA supplementation in older people. Each volunteer took 50 mg of the hormone every night

---

7   Ibid., 14.

8   Ibid., 14.

for three months before retiring. They reported an overall sense of well being, and both physically and emotionally, DHEA brought improvement.[9]

Each volunteer reported more energy, slept more soundly, were in better moods, and felt more relaxed and coped better than before taking the supplements. At last, evidence suggested the effectiveness of DHEA. It did for people what it did for animals and laboratory tests predicted it could and would do the same for humans.

Medical researcher, Dr. Richard Nestler, showed the DHEA's safety by administering 1,600 mg of the hormone to healthily young men every day for four weeks. There were no dangerous side effects. The positive results were excellent.[10]

The megadose of DHEA actually lowered cholesterol and decreased body fat. The more over weight the person was to start with, the greater weight loss was noted. These reports of Dr. Nestler are so very encouraging!

Studies now show that DHEA may be capable of preventing the onset of the dreaded disease of cancer. It seems to block the action of carcinogens, the substances that turn normal cells into dangerous cancer cells. It takes a long time for a normal cell to become cancerous. A carcinogen, such as ultraviolet light, tobacco, fats, alcohol, radiation, etc., comes into

---

9   Ibid., 17.

10 Ibid., 18.

contact with a cell and starts the change that brings about the growth of cancer.

A damaged cell can remain dormant for numerous years. Until it comes into contact with a "tumor promoter", or a substance that initiates further cellular division. After the damaged cell becomes cancerous, it will cause the growth of a tumor.

Dr. William Regelson, a professor of Medicine at the Medical College of Richmond, Virginia has evidence that DHEA slows down the action of these tumor promoters and halts the progression toward cancer. He relates "when carcinogens are awakened, they become active and the more active a carcinogen, the more mischief it can inflict. DHEA prevents cancer by intercepting these cellular wake-up calls."[11]

It is known that DHEA also acts as a antioxidant. This is important to know since it blocks the destructive effects of free radicals floating throughout the body.

In reference to cancer, it is so vastly momentous because DHEA may actually prevent cancer. Again this is due to its ability to block the effects of free radicals in the human system. This wonderful little hormone offers so much help for so many. Again, more research is needed before DHEA can be prescribed as a tool in the hands of physicians fighting cancer.

We do know that DHEA does boost the immune system. Medical science believes that the breakdown

---

11 Ibid., 40.

of the immune system is largely what allows cancer to take hold. Scientists believe that the key to cancer prevention is to find ways to bolster the immune function. DHEA does this very well.[12]

Remember your immune system does more than combat cancer cells. It is the human body's first line of defense against colds, flu, bacteria, viruses, fungi and infections of all kinds. As we become older, this wonderful system does not function as well as it did when we were much younger.

Dr. Regelson says, "Not only is there compelling evidence that DHEA can help us maintain a vigorous immune system, but research has also shown that it can take an aging, "broken" immune system and transform it into a young well-functioning system".[13]

DHEA has been linked with preventing heart disease. The best defense against heart disease includes consuming a high-fibre low-fat diet, reducing the intake of saturated fat and eating a variety of fresh fruits and vegetables daily. The American Heart Association recommends that people exercise five times a week for at least 30 minutes each workout session.

As early as the 1950's, scientists reported that heart disease patients had lower levels of DHEA. Since that time, it is known that patients with lower DHEA have higher levels of heart disease, especially among men.

---

12 Ibid., 42.

13 Ibid., 44.

Heart disease is a process in which deposits of thick, waxy fat deposits collect inside the arteries leading to the heart. These deposits are called plaque. The plaque consists of cholesterol, other fats, dead cells and other debris. The plaque causes a narrowing of the arteries which in some cases completely closes them.

A high fat-diet and a lack of exercise are the initial causes of blood thickening. This is a dangerous situation. Blood is to be thin and easily flowing through the circulatory system. When the blood is too thick, it an cause atherosclerosis. The danger of this is that the heart can be deprived of life-giving blood. When that happens, the heart goes into trauma resulting in a heart attack. Actual heart tissue will die when this occurs. A high fat diet is one of the major causes of this condition.

DHEA is known to shield us from atherosclerosis in several ways. It is a blood thinner, a cholesterol reducer and an antioxidant. Blood thinners are known to dissolve blood clots which will plug arteries and cause a heart attack.

Doctors recommend blood thinners on a regular basis from simple aspirin to more sophisticated drugs. Some of these actually cost several thousand dollars per injection. DHEA costs about fifteen cents per tablet.

There has been a great deal of study at the Medical College of Virginia which showed that DHEA thinned the blood and prevented additional clotting. A second study showed DHEA reduced clotting in people who had previously suffered from this condition. Dr. Regelson says that by "preventing excess blood clot formation, DHEA may protect against both heart disease and stroke."

DHEA has a cholesterol lowering effect. All of us know a little bit about cholesterol but the truth of the matter is many do not know how to keep our cholesterol at a normal level. High cholesterol raises the possibilities of a heart attack. It's just that simple!! Doctors tell us that our cholesterol should not be over 200. Readings over 200 are considered dangerous.

Dr. William Castelli, Director of the Harvard Medical School's Framingham Heart Study says that only real safe cholesterol level is 150 or below.[14] At that level heart attacks are very rare.

For some people it is very difficult to lower their cholesterol. At the same time, we need to be interested in what DHEA can do in lowering blood serum cholesterol.

In the 1980's, an indepth study was undertaken by the Medical College of Virginia where postmenopausal women were involved. After menopause, women have the identical risk as men do in having a heart attack or heart disease. DHEA was administered for a period of three months with the effects that cholesterol dropped by an average of 10 percent.[15] Dr. Regelson says that "this is significant given the fact that for every one

---

14 Ibid., 35.

15 Ibid., 36.

percent drop, there is a two percent drop in the risk of developing heart disease".[16]

Several scientists have spoken out on the role of DHEA and heart disease. Such men as Dr. Roger Blumenthal of John Hopkins University believes that the risk of heart attacks in both men and women is lowered by taking DHEA supplementation. However, we are cautioned not to assume that DHEA is a guaranteed heart medicine. Diet, exercise and supplementation all play a role in the prevention of heart disease.

Robert Jesse, M.D., Ph.D, of Medical College of Virginia has stated that, "There's a lot of information that indicates DHEA may have a protective role in the progression of heart disease". He further adds that it would be "reasonable to use DHEA supplements in older individuals to get levels back to those in youth."[17]

Please remember that to be free of heart disease requires a total life style of exercise, good nutrition, lots of good rest and proper supplementation. DHEA may become a part of this life style. You cannot and should not just depend on DHEA.

If you are a Christian and are still smoking, stop as soon as possible. You're opening the door for a demonic attack against you heart and your lungs.

Begin an exercise program and faithfully put it into practice at least five times a week for thirty or forty

---

16 Ibid., 36.

17 Ibid., 37.

minutes. Please see your doctor before starting an exercise program.

Change your diet and start eating more raw vegetables. Eat less meat but increase the amount of fruit in your diet. Stay away from fatty foods.

Make sure your blood pressure is within normal limits. Ask your doctor what you blood pressure should be and stay within that range.

Calm yourself down and let the peace of the Lord fill your mind. Meditation and prayer will help you relax and aid in the elimination of stress.

Make sure you take your antioxidants daily. Vitamin E and Vitamin C are so very necessary.

Do not take an aspirin a day unless your physician thinks it is wise for you.

Live a long life for the Lord! Psalm 91:6 promises us: "With a long life I will satisfy him, and let him behold My salvation." Take the promise God gives you and enjoy your life to the fullest with good health and lots of cheerful friends.

Eating To Win Beyond 2000 A.D.

# CHAPTER SIXTEEN

# THE CHOICE IS YOURS

As last we have come to the end of the book and now we need to make choices whether or not to apply the principles found with in this book. If we are to "Eat To Win" and become younger in the process, we have to start somewhere. Becoming younger through eating correctly is a slow process, requiring patience and diligence. This choice will require a great deal of personal discipline. All of us know that you can age over night, but to become healthier and younger in appearance will take a good amount of effort on your part to undo the damage which has been done by poor eating choices.

Wrong eating habits do not allow the cells to receive the nourishment necessary for living a full life. The cells and tissues must be supplied by nourishment from life food. As never before, we need to eat more raw vegetables and drink pure water, preferably steam distilled water. Cooking kills so many vitamins, minerals and enzymes. Processed foods do not enable us to sustain life at its peak. It is certain that processed foods will not supply the body with the nutrients necessary for regeneration. The aging process is excelled by eating dead processed foods. Only by eating live foods will the body obtain the living enzymes necessary for many vital functions of the body.

Let us never underestimate the importance of juicing. Juicing speeds up the time needed for body rejuvenation. Fresh raw vegetables made into juice helps speed this process. The body will react negatively if too much juice is taken in the early part of your health regime. So we need to understand this process and of the negative consequences, but above all, we must not become discourage. God works in mysterious ways so does Mother Nature. As we submit to this new style of living, we cannot be lot down. It takes time and effort to see the end results. There may be more to put right within your body than you first realized. As you comply with our new health program, you will see marvelous results. You will look and feel younger.

Do not live just to indulge your appetites and personal desires. Live a life with meaning, purpose and aim high in pursuing the best for yourself. Make a positive choice to eat correctly. Try cutting down on the amount of meat that you have been eating. Above all, stay away from pork. Pork is so very difficult to digest. A pig is an animal without sweat glands, except at the end of its nose. When the animal is slaughtered, the toxins are not expelled. When the flesh is cooked the toxins still remain and they finally make their way into your digestive system. Eating pork is like putting jet fuel into a Model T ford. Can you imagine what would happen? Just think what it does to your body. Stay away from pork and cut down on the amount of meat that you're eating. One must be very cautious also about eating deep fresh water fish. Such fish retain numerous toxic wastes and heavy metals such as lead and mercury.

Wrong living means living a life of mediocrity. Not only will wrong living affect the meaning of your life but even the quality of health. We cannot and must not live just for ourselves but if we don't take care of ourselves, who else will? You must take time and effort to care for your spiritual, mental and physical needs. If we don't take care of ourselves, we will soon become useless to ourselves and those that are a part of our world. There comes a time in each person's life that we give all we can of our physical, mental and spiritual qualities to the lives of others. As we give unto others we grow emotionally but above all we grow spiritually. As we study about the things of God and God's plan for eating, we will be utterly amazed how much we have gained. The new accumulated knowledge is like planting seeds. Seeds are totally worthless unless they are planted. Plant your new seeds of knowledge in helping others become better people.

It is like tithing which is God's plan for prosperity. Give 10 percent of what you make unto the work of the Lord and the law of sowing and reaping goes into effect and your abundance will greatly increase. Live right by following the Lord Jesus Christ. Learn how to eat right and so doing you will enjoy better health. Your life will be filled with new energy that can be used for the work of the Kingdom of God. We have to give in order to receive. "Give, and it will be given unto you", is the Lord's command. (Luke 6:38)

Wrong thinking will limit a person to a small little place in life. When we decide to think thoughts of goodness and purity our lives will be blessed beyond imagination. There is no truer saying than this: "As a man thinketh in his heart, so is he". This applies to all of us. Many diseases can be traced back to poor eating habits and poor thinking habits. By changing your life style, you will enjoy more of God's precious gift of Divine Health. It is possible. Start today with positive steps to improve your health and life. Only you can make the difference. Give yourself a real treat and Get Healthy!

# BIBLIOGRAPHY

**Atlas of Anatomy**, Marshall Cavendish Partworks, Ltd., London, U.K. 1993.

Ballentine, Rudolph., M.D. **Diet & Nutrition**, Pennsylvania, The Himalayan International Institute, 1989.

Berkow, Robert, M.D. **The Merck Manual**, Merck Shart & Dohme Research Laboratories, Rahway, New Jersey, 1987.

Bragg, Paul C. N.D., Ph.D. **Miracle of Fasting**, Health Science, Santa Barbara, California, 1981.

Buchman, Dian Dincin. **Herbal Medicine**, Gramercy Publishing Co., New York, 1979.

Dhillon, Sukhraj S., Ph.D. **Health, Happiness, & Longevity**, Japan Publications, New York, 1983.

Douillard, John. **Body, Mind And Sport**, Harmony Books, New York, 1994.

Dox, Ida G., Ph.D., John Belloni, Ph.D. and Gilbert M. Eisner, M.D. **The Harper Collins Illustrated Medical Dictionary**, Harper Collins Publishers, New York, 1993.

Guyton, Arthur C. **Basic Human Physiology**, W. R.

Saunders Co., Philadelphia, Pennsylvania, 1977.

Jensen, Dr. Bernard. **Slender Me Naturally**, Bernard Jensen Enterprises, Escondido, California, 1986.

_ _ _ _ _ _ _ _. **Tissue Cleansing Through Bowel Management**, Bernard Jensen Enterprises, Escondido, California, 1981.

_ _ _ _ _ _ _ _. **Food Healing For Man**, Bernard Jensen Enterprises, Escondido, California, 1983.

Kloss, Jethro. **Back To Eden**, Back To Eden Publishing Co., California, 1992.

Marti, James and Andrea Hine. **Alternative Health Medicine Encyclopedia**, Visible Ink Press, Detroit, Michigan, 1955.

Michaud, Ellen; Sara J. Henry; Brenda Becker, Michael Castleman and Mathew Hoffman. **The Complete Book of Natural & Medicinal Cures**, Rodale Press, Emmaus, Pennsylvania, 1994.

Miller, Benjamin F. and Claire Brockman Keane. **Encyclopedia and Dictionary of Medicine, Nursing, and Allied Health**, W. B. Saunders Company, Philadelphia, Pennsylvania, 1983.

**Mosby's Medical Dictionary**, Mosby Year Book, Inc., St. Louis, Missouri, 1994.

Murray, Michael N.D., and Joseph Pezzorno, N.D. **Encyclopedia of Natural Medicine**, Prima Publishing, Rocklin, California, 1991.

O'Brien, Jim. **Why Everyone's Talking About DHEA**, Globe Communications Corp., Boca Raton, Florida, 1997.

Oppenheim, Michael, M.D. **The Man's Health Book**, Prentice-Hall Inc., Englewood Cliffs, New Jersey, 1994.

Register, V. and L. Sonnenberg "The Vegetarian Diet". **Journal of American Diet Association**, 1973

Ritchason, Jack, N.D. **The Little Herb Encyclopedia**, Woodland Health Books, Pleasant Grove, Utah, 1995.

Sahelian, Ray, M.D. **DHEA**, Avery Publishing Group, Garden City Park, New York, 1996.

Schumacher, Teresa & Toni Schumacher Lund. **Cleansing the Body and the Colon for a Happier and Healthier You**, St. George, Utah, 1994.

Wade, Carlson. **Magic Minerals**, Parker Publishing Company, New York, 1986.

_ _ _ _ _ _ _ _. **Nutritional Healers**, Parker Publishing Company, New York, 1987.

Walker, Dr. N. W., D.Sc. **Become Younger**, O'Sullivan Woodside & Co, Phoenix, Arizona, 1984.

Notes

Notes

Notes